KETO IN 28

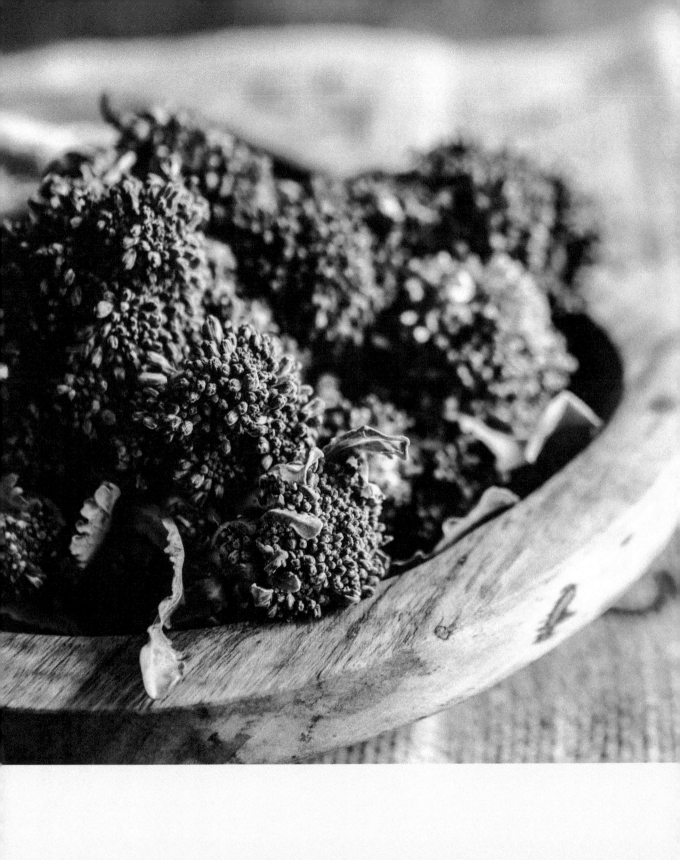

MICHELLE HOGAN

KETO IN 28

The Ultimate

LOW-CARB, HIGH-FAT

Weight-Loss Solution

SONOMA
PRESS

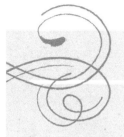

QUICK START GUIDE

Keto in 28 is a comprehensive yet simple guide to getting into ketosis and losing weight. Whether you've experimented with a ketogenic diet before or have never heard of it until now, this book will motivate you with a reasonable 28-day plan. My own personal experience with the keto lifestyle will help you get through cravings, the "carb flu," exercise, and the fads that keep you buying products you don't need to "go keto." If you're thinking, "Oh no, another diet," don't worry. There are no points, portion-controlling containers, calorie counters, other apparatus, or gimmicks. Stick with me and you'll be amazed at the results.

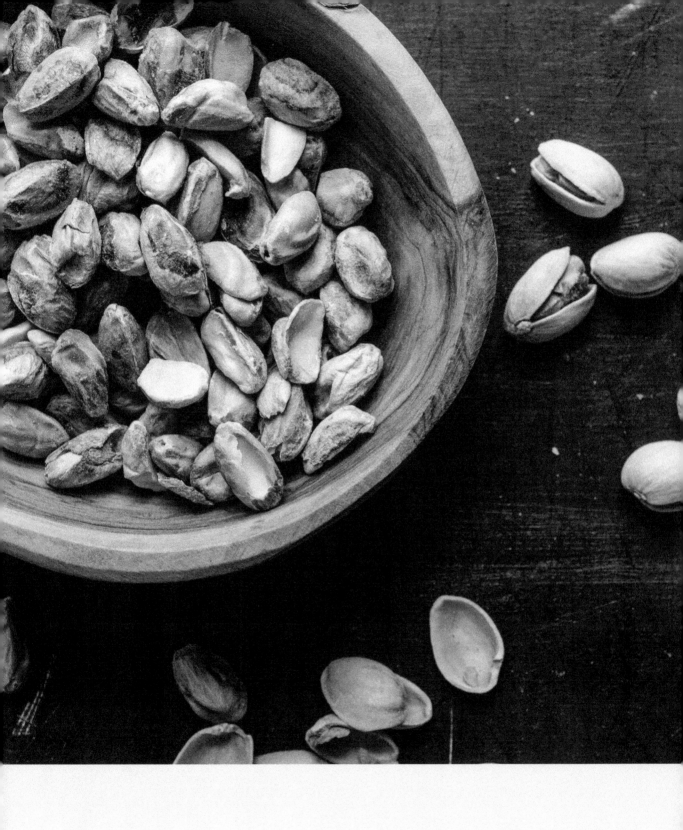

CONTENTS

FOREWORD

Poor dietary habits and a sedentary lifestyle are contributing factors to the obesity epidemic that's on the rise in the United States. According to the Centers of Disease Control and Prevention, more than one-third of U.S. adults are obese. There are so many diets out there today that promise and promote so many things; it's challenging to know which diet may be suited for you? As a Registered Dietitian, I have worked with diverse populations, requiring different medical nutrition therapy prescriptions, including the ketogenic diet. While some may be skeptical about the restrictiveness of ketogenic diet, it is important to note that studies have proven this way of eating to be helpful and safe for significantly overweight and obese individuals. At first it might seem counterintuitive to eat this way—consuming lots of fat—but it's easily possible to get all the nutrition your body needs. When starting any new diet program, it's important to discuss your plan with your doctor. This is especially true if you are starting keto and currently taking any medications for diabetes of high blood pressure.

The ketogenic diet consists of high-fat, moderate protein diet with very low intake of carbohydrates. The restriction of carbohydrates causes your glycogen (stored carbohydrates) level to drop and the body goes into ketosis. When your body is in the state of ketosis, it creates ketones. Research has found that during very low carbohydrate intake, the accumulation of ketone bodies causes a harmless physiological state, known as dietary ketosis, in which your body burns fat reserves for energy. Dietary ketosis is often, and wrongly, confused with ketoacidosis, a condition harmful to diabetics.

The ketogenic diet is relatively easy to follow if you have an outline of what steps you need to take. In this book, Michelle did a wonderful job outlining the diet, meal by meal, for 28 days, making it simple for anyone to follow. She lays out exactly what you need to succeed. Michelle is with you every step of the way. The recipes included are delicious, nutritious, and very filling.

Michelle also shares with you her very own successful story with keto. After many failed attempts of struggling with her fluctuating weight, she took the initiative to take control of her life and try something different. She found balance following the ketogenic diet and incorporating physical activity and has lost more than 100 pounds. I understand the frustration of wanting to lose weight and keep it off, as many of my clients find themselves in this predicament. There are many diets and weight loss products on the market, making it difficult to know which one is right for you. I think the key to weight loss success is finding something that fits you and your needs. The ketogenic diet is one way to kick-start your journey to successful weight loss.

—Susan Zogheib, RD
susueats.com

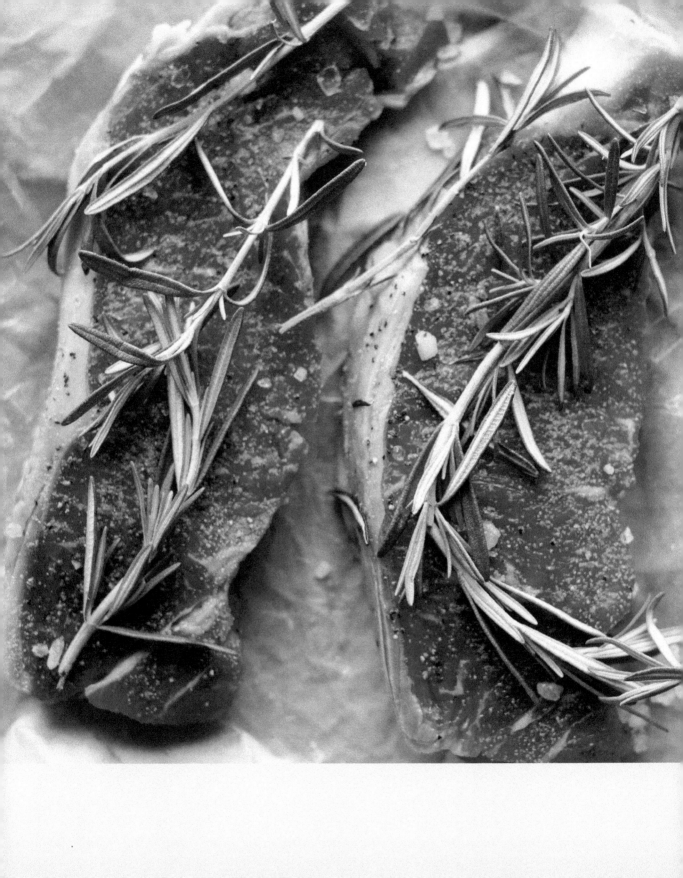

INTRODUCTION

MY STORY WITH KETO

In 2009, I found myself not only carrying a wonderful new baby (my seventh) in my arms, but also about 100 additional pounds. I distinctly remember the day I caught sight of my rear end in the mirror after taking a shower. I was absolutely stunned. This was not the me I remembered—even after kids five and six. I had to do something to be healthier and fit into pants I already owned. I was tired of choosing between buying clothes in bigger and bigger sizes or suffering with a waistband that cut into my stomach.

I didn't know where to begin. Over the years that followed, I tried all sorts of diets, but none for very long. I hate being starve-yourself-and-then-eat-everything-you-see hungry, and I'm not a huge fan of salad. I would eat it, but lettuce, a few anemic tomatoes, and a cucumber did not shield me from hunger. After researching on numerous blogs about various diets, I discovered the ketogenic approach. It took me almost a year to make the transition, but once I did, the results were well worth my efforts. I was comfortable wearing a bathing suit. Muscle definition in my thighs and calves was visible for the first time in my life. I could walk a mile, then run a 5K, without being winded. I had more energy, slept better, and didn't want to sit on the couch watching TV. Getting myself to sit for an extended period to read a book took more effort than going for a walk. That had never happened before!

Starting a new, healthy lifestyle can be intimidating. It can also be a little annoying—especially if you think you eat pretty well already. Once you get past these or any other resistance that you might be feeling, you'll be ready to give yourself this new beginning. Taking this chance promises you success if you take the keto lifestyle seriously and play by this book.

Part 1 of *Keto in 28*, "The Keto Diet—A Closer Look," begins with a keto primer that acquaints you with the basics of your new lifestyle. It coaches you on what to expect and gives you an overview of foods to embrace and those to avoid. You'll also get answers to some frequently asked questions. This is the section of the book where you'll also find out how to stock your kitchen and plan your meals ahead. Part 1 ends with five encouraging ideas to help you start or maintain your exercise program.

Part 2, "28-Day Meal Plan," plots out the first four weeks of your keto lifestyle. It provides you with simple, quick, and budget-friendly ways to incorporate the diet into your life—instead of making your life revolve around your diet. Many recipes contain five ingredients or fewer and take less than 40 minutes to prepare. This is also where you'll be introduced to shopping lists and snacks.

Keto in 28 is designed with a busy person in mind. You don't have to dread searching for odd, exotic ingredients. Of course, if you like to cook and want to experiment—go for it! However, your weight-loss success does not depend on camping out in the kitchen. It will be simple to keep your fridge and pantry stocked. "What's for dinner?" will become an easy question to answer. As soon as you hit week 4, you're greeted with the chapter "Beyond Your First 28 Days" to help you stay on track.

The 122 recipes in part 3 are sprinkled with a variety of useful tips:

- **A CLOSER LOOK** tips offer a deeper profile of one of the recipe's ingredients that digs into its health benefits.
- **TRY INSTEAD** tips suggest ingredient substitutions.
- **KITCHEN HACK** tips tell you how to save time or money.

In addition to standard nutrition information, each recipe includes its own macronutrient ratio.

A ketogenic lifestyle encourages you to reduce the amount of carbs you take in each day and replace them with foods that have few or no carbs. One of the great things about going keto is being able to indulge your love for things that are off-limits for many other diets—like bacon fat and butter—and figuring out ways to use them to flavor foods you want to eat. Bacon fat drizzled over salad greens is an awesome salad dressing. Avocados are a great lunch when eaten whole out of their rind and salted—or scooped out on a plate with a couple of fresh eggs fried in bacon fat or butter on top.

Changing what you eat, how you eat, and the way you think of food can be quite a challenge. However, making those changes can be well worthwhile and transformative. *Keto in 28* shows you how to implement small changes over a period of 28 days. You'll be pleased by how much you can accomplish in that short period of time.

PART I

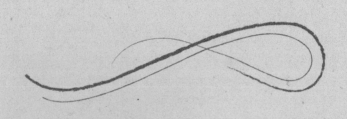

THE
KETO DIET—
A CLOSER LOOK

BEGINNING A KETOGENIC DIET is pretty straightforward. Your goal is to put your body into *ketosis*. This is the process in which your body starts to produce *ketones*, which are by-products of the fat-burning process. You need to start eliminating as many carbohydrates as possible, particularly those from high-sugar and -starch sources. The keto lifestyle is effective for two basic reasons: ketosis helps you burn more fat, and by simply eating more fat and protein, you end up eating less. Eating more fat also encourages your body to burn more fat while you're resting. The idea of eating fat and losing weight can take some getting used to. That's the purpose of chapters 1 and 2, "Your Keto Primer" and "28 Days to Keto Success," respectively. They provide the foundation you need to understand the value of this new dietary lifestyle.

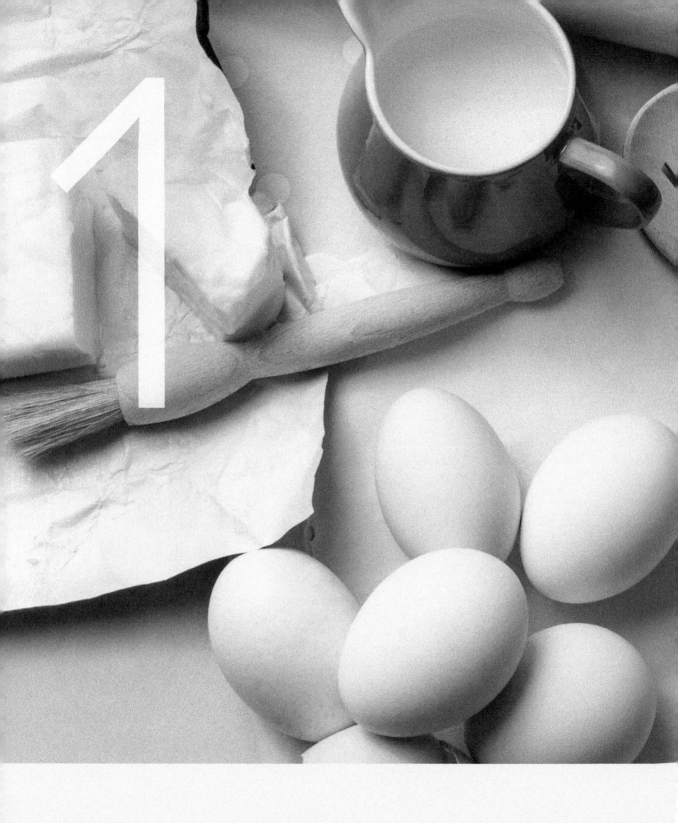

YOUR KETO PRIMER

Ketogenic diets are nothing new. Historically, humans have been driven to consume sugar, which used to be harder to find. Now, sugar is everywhere and in everything. It's a major contributor to weight gain and obesity.

Getting your body to rid itself of excess blood sugar and glycogen is the key to entering ketosis. *Glycogen* is the main form of energy storage in most animals. Once in ketosis, your body will not only start to burn off fat, but it will also begin to "power up" your brain. While the science behind this "powering up" of the brain is not yet readily accessible to the general public, many people report feeling clearer and more focused after being on a ketogenic diet.

This primer explains the finer details of keto, including macronutrient ratios, what you should expect from following the keto lifestyle, and the possibility of experiencing keto flu. You'll also learn about what you should and should not eat (and drink) in order to get the greatest benefits from your new eating lifestyle. Finally, you'll find answers to five questions that every keto eater can answer.

WHAT IS KETO?

Keto is a very low-carbohydrate diet. *Carbohydrates* are organic compounds that include sugars. Your body needs *glucose*, which is a simple sugar. Glucose helps your brain work and gets energy to muscles, like your heart, and to your liver. The amount of sugar you need depends on your metabolism, energy level, and body size. If you have more glucose than you need at one time, your body stores it to use later as fat.

The low-carb diet is the basis for others such as Atkins, Paleo, and parts of the South Beach diet. They all rely on consuming minimal amounts of sugar (carbs) in order to put your body in the right metabolic state to lose weight. Most proponents of a ketogenic diet don't believe in counting calories because most of your calories will come from foods that will not cause a spike in insulin production, as can happen in a high-carb diet.

In addition to discouraging the consumption of most grain-based items and legumes, a keto diet is also essentially gluten-free, simply because most bread and grain products (the products that contain gluten) are eliminated. Often gluten-free products are loaded with extra sugars to give them the mouthfeel they are lacking by not having gluten to hold them together. In general, if you're going to have a cheat day, you will probably find "real food," rather than processed food items, most satisfying.

WHAT TO EXPECT

What results should you expect from a ketogenic diet? Before starting any diet, it's important to realize that you are still *you*. Lose weight because you want to be healthier and feel better about yourself if you are overweight. If you're struggling to walk up stairs, losing weight will help you with that. If you want to run a marathon, losing weight will help you achieve that goal. Take each day in the 28-day plan slowly, and remember that going on the journey is as important as achieving your objective.

KETO GLOSSARY

Understanding these terms clearly will contribute to your success with *Keto in 28*.

AMINO ACIDS are the building blocks of the proteins the body needs to do everything from build muscle to grow hair and nails.

ANABOLIC HORMONES stimulate protein synthesis, insulin production, and muscle growth.

BMR (BASAL METABOLIC RATE) is the amount of energy expended while the body is at rest.

CARBOHYDRATES are organic compounds occurring in foods and living tissues and include sugars, starch, and cellulose. They can be broken down to release energy in the animal body.

CYTOKINES are a broad and loose category of small proteins that are released by cells and affect the behavior of other cells.

ELECTROLYTES are minerals in your blood and other body fluids that affect the amount of water in your body, the acidity of your blood (pH), your muscle function, and other important processes.

GLUCOSE is a simple sugar that is considered to be an important energy source in living organisms and is a component of carbohydrates.

GLYCOGEN is a substance deposited in bodily tissues as a store of carbohydrates.

KETOGENIC or KETO relates to the production of ketones in the body.

KETONES are any of a class of organic compounds that burn fat when the body can't burn glucose for energy.

KETOSIS is the act of creating ketones while burning fat for energy.

LEAN MASS WEIGHT or LEAN BODY MASS is the amount your body weighs without fat.

MACRONUTRIENTS are substances such as fat or protein that your body requires in large amounts.

METABOLISM is the process by which your body converts the food and drink you consume into energy. During this complex biochemical process, calories in food and beverages are combined with oxygen to release the energy your body needs to function.

UNDERSTANDING RATIOS

Your *macronutrient ratio* consists of the amounts of fat, carbs, and protein that you should take in daily in relation to one another. Each recipe in this book lists these ratios in a relationship of fat to protein. For example, the very first recipe in chapter 5, "Breakfast," is Creamy Cinnamon Breakfast Pudding (page 64). Its macronutrient breakdown is Fat 75% / Carbs 7% / Protein 18%. Its fat-to-protein ratio is 2:1.

Two factors that influence your macronutrient level are lean mass weight (what you weigh without any fat) and activity level. Here are some examples of the latter:

- SEDENTARY: most office jobs, very little or no exercise (light walking)

- LIGHTLY ACTIVE: 1 to 3 times a week, light exercise such as light cardio (walking, light cycling)

- MODERATELY ACTIVE: 3 to 5 times a week (moderate cardio and muscle training)

- VERY ACTIVE: 5 or more times a week (hard exercise, intense cardio and muscle training at fitness level)

- ATHLETES / BODYBUILDERS: daily exercise at professional level (high-intensity exercise)

Following is a basic formula from the Keto Diet Blog to help you work out your macronutrient ratio. Say you weigh 160 pounds and have 30% body fat. Your lean mass weight would be calculated as follows:

160 lbs – 30% = 112 lbs

Multiply the result by 0.6 to determine the *minimum* grams of protein you should consume:

112 × 0.6 = 67 g of protein

Multiply the result by 1 to determine the *maximum* grams of protein you should consume:

112 × 1 = 112 g of protein

Therefore, your daily protein intake should be between 67 and 112 g.

If you're unsure of your body fat percentage, the Keto Diet Blog also includes instructions for making this calculation.

Here's what to expect as you follow *Keto in 28*:

1. Fewer cravings.

A ketogenic diet will gradually keep you from wanting bad foods. Believe me! I was a sweet-a-holic. I loved anything with sugar: doughnuts in particular or any kind of cake. I still love to look at that stuff; I just don't want it anymore. I know a couple of superior bakeries, and I will shop there for my friends and family for their birthdays. I greatly admire the effort that goes into making some of these treats. But my desire to eat them is really gone. When I occasionally give into temptation, a bite or two is enough. My body doesn't feel the need to gorge like it used to. It's very strange for me, because I will still watch pastry TV shows on the Food Network and think, "That looks delicious." But I don't want to eat it.

2. Reduced appetite.

Not only will eating ketogenically kill your cravings, it will bring down your appetite as well because carbs stimulate your appetite. Eating a low-carb diet keeps your appetite in check so you eat fewer calories and lose weight, naturally. Write down what you eat for a few days. Don't go hungry, but see what you eat. I'll bet you'll be surprised by how few calories you take in.

3. Rapid weight loss—especially in the beginning.

Why? Well, it will be mostly water weight right at the beginning, but you know what? Many "experts" say that water-weight loss doesn't count, but in reality, it does. Your body holds onto excess water when you eat too many carbs. You'll lose weight faster than other dieters—particularly those on low-fat diets. In the beginning, this is due to water-weight loss, but as you continue, you'll see a more rapid weight loss due to ketosis fat-burning. If you maintain the lifestyle, you'll keep it off longer, too.

4. Eat all the fat you want, and lose more weight.

Yeah. It's that amazing. Do not, under any circumstances, eat low-fat or reduced-fat anything. Eat butter. Eat full-fat cheese and milk. Fry your eggs in lard. Eating a diet that is 70 percent fat, 25 percent protein, and only 15 percent carbs will also raise your HDL (good) cholesterol and decrease your triglycerides according to a 2003 study in *The Journal of Pediatrics*.

5. Decreased risk for metabolic syndrome, high blood pressure, and high blood sugar (and type 2 diabetes).

High blood sugar alone isn't type 2 diabetes; however, prolonged exposure to high blood sugar can cause your pancreas to reduce its production of insulin, causing type 2 diabetes. Basically, in type 2 diabetes, your body becomes desensitized to the presence of sugar. If you have these conditions already, it's highly likely that they will be greatly reduced or disappear altogether.

6. More muscle equals less fat.

By consuming muscle meat and protein, you are building muscle—and therefore increasing your metabolism. Protein is *anabolic* and used for building new cells, like muscle. Muscles require more energy to move, so just by building more muscle mass, you are burning more energy and raising your metabolism. Bonus! According to McKinley Health Center at the University of Illinois at Urbana-Champaign, some people have genetics to thanks for having higher metabolic rates than others, but it's important to consider muscle mass when determining your BMR. Muscle is more active and demands more energy than fat, so if you have a higher percentage of muscle compared to fat, you will have a higher BMR.

7. Increased gut health.

We all hear about probiotics and improving the bacteria in our gut, but how can eating ketogenically help with that? Sugars and processed foods cause inflammation in your intestinal tract. When you combine carbs, processed foods, and stress, tiny perforations form in your intestinal walls, and waste products and digestive acids that shouldn't leave your intestinal tract end up leaking out. According to Harvard Health Publications, the rush of blood sugar you get when eating a meal or snack of highly refined carbohydrates (white bread, white rice, French fries, sugar-laden soda, etc.) increases your level of inflammatory messengers called cytokines.

FACING THE FLU

After a few days on a low-carb or ketogenic diet, you may find yourself fighting something called the carb flu. Basically, this is your body's way of recalculating your metabolism. All of a sudden, you are not processing the foods your body is used to processing, and you are processing higher quantities of other foods.

Think of your GPS when you turn somewhere unplanned. Instead of taking in the foods that are familiar to your body, you are sending in nutrients that your body has to "think" about and use a lot of energy to process. This is a good thing! This means it's working. But, it also means you may feel a little more tired than usual. You might find yourself a little foggier in the brain than normal. You may get a few headaches or even feel nauseous. Drinking a little fresh ginger and lemon steeped in hot water can help with that.

Your body is full of enzymes that are waiting for those carbs you usually eat, but they aren't coming in. Now your body has to create new enzymes that will burn fat for fuel instead of carbs. The transition is called *the low-carb* or *ketosis flu*.

Give it a few days—or even a week or two—to sort itself out. In that time, continue eating ketogenically, but if you don't feel like doing hard-core exercise, don't. Take walks instead, ride a bike, or play. Some people find that days two and three can be challenging, and scheduling these days to fall on a weekend (or other day with low activity) can be beneficial.

Remember, especially as you're starting out, to keep replenishing your water: tap, distilled, mineral, or sparkling. Drink bone broth (chicken or beef). Eat fats such as avocados and some butter (hold the bread and potatoes). Try not to overeat protein if you're feeling very sick, as doing so can make it worse before it gets better.

Fatty meats and cheeses can help ease the transition and ensure that your body doesn't convert the protein to glucose. If you have high blood pressure or cholesterol, you may want to consult with your doctor first.

You are teaching your body how to eat in a whole new way!

WHAT TO EAT AND WHAT NOT TO EAT

On the keto diet, you'll consume calories primarily from fats and then from proteins. Once you determine your correct macronutrient ratio, you can figure out how much of each type of food to eat. When in doubt, go heavy on the fat and vegetables and light on the protein.

Foods to Eat

These are the foods to eat all the time in liberal quantities.

Avocado Avocados have more potassium than bananas, and they are loaded with fiber. They contain oleic acid, which is a monounsaturated fat that reduces inflammation.

Cheese and Dairy (full fat) Always choose the full-fat versions of yogurt (plain), butter, cheeses, and milk. Be wary of using too much dairy to replace carbs, as you might upset your stomach at first.

Cruciferous Vegetables Broccoli, cauliflower, kale, and cabbages are widely considered to be anticancerous. They're also low in carbs and fill you up. Cauliflower makes a great substitute for mashed potatoes.

Ghee (pronounced "gee") Ghee is clarified butter and is rich in oil-soluble vitamins A and E. It's rich in K_2 and conjugated linoleic acid (an antioxidant with antiviral properties) and is beneficial to the immune system.

Greens Leafy green vegetables such as spinach, kale, Swiss chard, lettuces, and arugula are excellent sources of fiber, minerals, and vitamins. They might also offer protection against heart disease, cancer, and diabetes.

Fatty Meats Look for chicken and other poultry with the skin still on, ground beef or pork that's 80/20, and other cuts of meat such as rib eye steaks.

Squashes Squash cooked almost any way is a good way to get a starchy feel out of a low-carb vegetable. As a bonus, squash is full of antioxidants and plenty of vitamins.

Keep these foods off the menu for the first 28 days.

Fruits Fruits have a lot of sugar. Berries like blueberries and blackberries are fine to eat in small quantities.

Foods That Grow Below Ground If it's a carrot, potato, parsnip, or another "root" vegetable, you should probably avoid it for the time being.

Processed Foods From American cheese to anything that comes in a box, just stay away from processed meals. Buy the actual food item, and you'll find it much easier to stick to your plan.

IS IT KETO-FRIENDLY?

BARS such as Atkins, Luna, and others claim to be high in protein and low in carbs. Usually, they don't fill you up and have more carbs than you need and way more calories than they're worth for the serving. It's better to avoid these.

BEEF JERKY is often touted as one of the best snacking options for keto eaters, but too much protein can be quickly turned into glucose. Watch for nitrates and sugars.

HARD-BOILED EGGS make a perfect snack.

PEANUT BUTTER can be a great low-carb, higher-protein option, especially for snacks. However, be wary of eating too much or buying brands with added sugar, which can increase the carbs.

PEPPERONI pairs nicely with bites of cheese and fresh tomato and basil. Always try to choose meats (jerky, pepperoni) that are nitrite- and nitrate-free.

PORK RINDS are an excellent salty snack. Try not to go "crazy," but even if you do, this treat should not make you feel guilty.

FOODS TO EAT AND AVOID

	EAT	AVOID
Fruits	Blueberries, Cranberries, Strawberries (occasionally), Apples (occasionally), Watermelon (occasionally)	Peaches, Plums, Melons, Citrus (except for lemon in water and lime in guacamole)
Vegetables	Spinach, Kale, Broccoli, Cauliflower, Lettuces (all sorts), Sweet potatoes (occasionally, as meal replacement), Kohlrabi, Fennel, Avocado, Squashes, Tomatoes, Green peppers, Hot peppers, Onions, Garlic, Asparagus, Mushrooms, Cucumbers	Carrots, Potatoes, Parsnips, Turnips, Rutabagas
Grains		Avoid all
Dairy	Whole milk, Whole-fat cheese (cow, goat, sheep), Butter, 2 to 4 percent–fat yogurt (sometimes it's hard to find 4 percent), Cottage cheese, Whole ricotta, Buttermilk, Sour cream, Whipping cream	All reduced-fat or skim products
Nuts and Seeds	Macadamias, Walnuts, Coconuts, Pecans, Brazil nuts, and Almonds are best. Nut and seed flours are okay for some breadings and "baked" goods, but only in moderation. Almond flour is good as a thickening agent if needed.	Chestnuts, Cashews, Pistachios (eat minimally; they are higher in carbs than other nuts)

	EAT	AVOID
Fats and Oils	Avocado oil, Olive oil, Coconut oil, Flaxseed oil, Palm oil (sustainably grown and made), Beef tallow, Chicken fat, Lard, Bacon fat, Mayonnaise (made with olive oil). Try to get organic, extra-virgin when possible, but if cost is a factor, even lower-cost olive oil is better than canola oil.	Canola oil, Vegetable oil, Safflower oil, Margarine, Butter blends, Crisco or "hydrogenated" cooking oils
Spices and Herbs	Sea salt, Black pepper, Basil, Cayenne pepper, Chili powder, Cilantro, Cinnamon, Cumin, Oregano, Parsley, Rosemary, Sage, Thyme, Turmeric	Premade mixes because they have added sugar.
Sugar and Sweetener	Stevia	Aspartame, Xylitol, Sucralose, Sugar
Protein	Wild-caught salmon, Halibut, Cod, Flounder, Lobster, Crab, Scallops, Tuna, Chicken, Beef, Lamb, Venison, Bison, Bacon (uncured), Ham, (uncured), Sausages	Tilapia, Farm-raised salmon, Cured deli meats, Cured hot dogs, Cured bacon, all nitrates in meat

5 QUESTIONS EVERY KETO EATER CAN ANSWER

This is not a quiz, but you'll come up with your own answers to these questions as you work your way through *Keto in 28*.

1. How long does it take for a person to go into ketosis?

It will take anywhere from 2 to 7 days to go into ketosis, depending on how low you go with your carbs. If you restrict your carbs to 20 grams or less, you will go into ketosis much faster than someone who limits themselves to 50 grams or less.

2. What are ketostix, and how do I use them?

Ketostix are usually used by pregnant women during prenatal visits and type 1 diabetics to detect the presence of ketones in their urine. They work in essentially the same way that pH strips work, changing color based on the level of ketones detected in your urine. Ketostix can help motivate you with clearly visible results, but shouldn't be considered the ultimate determination of how this diet is working for you. How you feel and the weight coming off are much more important.

WHAT ABOUT ALCOHOL?

It's a good idea to avoid alcohol entirely during the 28-day plan. After that, you can work it back into your meal plan. Red wine is a low-carb choice, and there are a number of liquors (unflavored) that have zero carbs. However, drinking alcohol can also cause your metabolism to slow down. Your willpower could suffer, too, and eating more before bedtime may be easier to rationalize. If you're committed to going keto, take at least a week or two to detox your body fully before adding alcohol back in.

3. Constipation. How do I stop it?

Constipation can happen on a ketogenic diet. Experiment with these remedies to relieve the discomfort:

- Drink a glass of water every hour or so.
- Eat a tablespoon of coconut oil.
- Eat fibrous veggies and more greens with each meal.
- Stop eating a lot of nuts if you are doing so.
- Add chia, flax, or hemp seeds into your diet (in yogurts and smoothies).
- Drink coffee or tea.
- Take a magnesium supplement.

Important: Try these solutions one at a time, as needed, rather than all at once.

4. Why do I need to drink so much water?

Being in ketosis helps your body eliminate water rapidly. This means you have to replace the water and everything that goes along with it. Coconut water and bone broth will help you replace your electrolytes and can also relieve symptoms of the carb flu.

5. What do I eat when I'm traveling?

You eat the same things you would eat otherwise. If you're eating out, you'll find it simple to eat the chicken and fish dishes, not fried, and with a side salad—no potatoes please! At a burger joint, have the burger "open-faced" over lettuce, smothered in cheese, mushrooms, and onions, and eat it with a fork and knife. Find yourself hungry at a gas station? Go with pork rinds or beef jerky. Some also have yogurt. A grocery store is your friend. If you carry a clean pocket knife, you can grab an avocado, slice it down the middle, remove the pit, salt it, and eat it straight out of the rind with a spoon. Want a salad? Grab a salad in the bag from the grocery store and some rotisserie chicken pieces to toss in with it—instant salad. Are your friends ordering a pizza? Eat the toppings off, and leave the crust behind. Grandma's making her famous pasta dish? Ask if you can have just the meat sauce and cheese in a bowl. I do this all the time—it's a little like "pasta" stew, but seriously yummy.

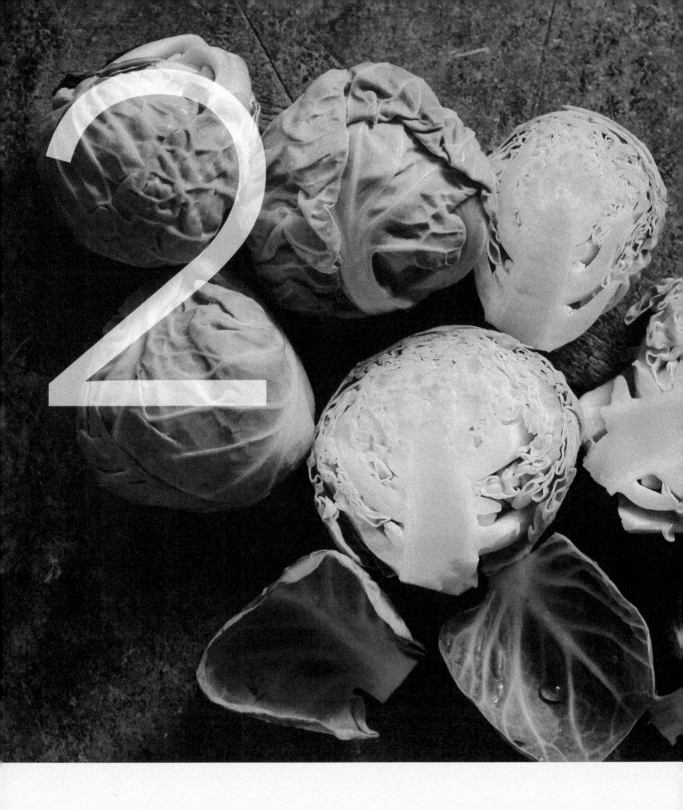

28 DAYS TO KETO SUCCESS

A ketogenic lifestyle is not hard to maintain. Just eat the right foods in almost any quantity you want. Don't even worry about ratios in the first couple of days. Why? Well, if you're used to eating breads, grains, and starches, you might feel a little deprived. But if you can eat a roast chicken for dinner and steak and eggs for lunch, without guilt, you're going to feel a lot better about losing out on garlic bread at dinner. Once your body starts to adapt to keto, you can concentrate on the ratios and quantities of what you're eating.

This chapter gets you that much closer to starting your new lifestyle. Here, you'll learn how to stock your pantry and which spices to keep on hand. Concerned about kitchen tools? You'll be glad to know that very few are required. We'll explore the easiest ways to plan ahead, and last but not least, you'll be reminded of how important it is to exercise.

PANTRY ESSENTIALS

Stocking your pantry is crucial to your success. If you don't want to have to shop each day for your meal, keeping and organizing your pantry will make each day's meals easy to prepare. The best advice one can get when it comes to shopping is to stick to the list and to shop at the outside edge of the store—that's where the produce and protein are. If you're super busy and don't want to be tempted by in-store items (and you can afford it), find out if your local store offers delivery service or, at least, a shopping service where you can pick up the groceries after work; many urban stores do.

Each week of the 28-day plan offers a comprehensive shopping list, which details everything you need for the week. Once you've completed the 28 days, keeping items from the list below on hand can make creating your own meal plan (or throwing together a quick dinner) very simple.

Allspice, ground

Almond flour

Almonds

Anchovy fillets

Applesauce, unsweetened

Arrowroot

Baking powder

Baking soda

Basil, dried

Black pepper, freshly ground

Blueberries, dried

Brazil nuts

Broth, beef

Broth, chicken

Cashews

Cayenne pepper, ground

Chia seeds

Chili powder

Chipotle peppers in adobo

Cinnamon, ground

Coconut, unsweetened shredded

Coriander, ground

Cranberries, dried

Cumin, ground

Curry paste

Curry powder

Egg white protein powder

Fish and chicken, canned organic
    (for quick meals)

Fish sauce

Flax meal, regular, golden

Flax seeds

Ghee

Ginger, ground

Hazelnuts (filberts), chopped

Hot sauce, such as Tabasco

Lemon extract

Macadamia nuts

Milk, almond, unsweetened

Milk, coconut

Mustard, Dijon

Mustard, grainy

Nutmeg, ground

Oil, coconut

Oil, extra-virgin olive

Oil, sesame

Oil, walnut

Olives, canned or jarred

Oregano, dried

Paprika, ground

Peanut butter, natural

Peanuts

Pecans

Pistachios

Pumpkin seeds

Sambal oelek

Sea salt

Sesame seeds

Soy sauce

Stevia

Sunflower seeds

Taco seasoning

Tahini

Tomatoes, sun-dried, packed in oil

Vanilla extract, pure

Vinegar, apple cider

Vinegar, balsamic

Vinegar, sherry

Walnuts

Worcestershire sauce

THE KETO SPICE RACK

Herbs and spices aren't just a great way to add zip to your meals; they can also help you in your efforts to lose weight. Different spices and herbs have distinct properties and nutrients. Cinnamon, for example, reduces blood sugar levels and carb cravings. Mustard seed can boost your metabolism, as can cayenne pepper. Turmeric has major antioxidant qualities, and many other herbs and spices can tip the scales in your favor.

Anise, ground (for a fantastic
  licorice flavor)

Basil, dried

Black pepper, freshly ground

Cayenne pepper, ground

Celery seed

Cinnamon, ground

Coriander, ground

Cumin, ground

Dill, dried

Garlic powder

Ginger, ground

Marjoram, ground

Mustard seed

Oregano (the oil of which
has amazing healing
properties), dried

Salt, preferably sea
(iodized)

Thyme, dried

Turmeric, ground

KITCHEN TOOLS

You don't need a bunch of kitchen tools to make great food. With some simple pots and pans and basic tools, you have everything you need. Avoid nonstick cookware, and buy cast iron when you can. Cast iron can be made nonstick with proper seasoning, and it adds a little extra iron to the food you eat.

HEALTH BENEFITS OF HERBS AND SPICES

Many of the herbs and spices that you'll use as part of following *Keto in 28* have impressive health benefits.

CILANTRO is high in antioxidants, potassium, and vitamins A, C, and K. This pretty dark green herb can help reduce cholesterol levels, support a healthy cardiovascular system, and reduce the risk of Alzheimer's disease. It also has a distinct anise or licorice flavor and is a good source of antioxidants and phytonutrients.

TARRAGON contains iron, calcium, potassium, and vitamin A. It has been used as a folk medicine for stimulating appetite, and it can support the cardiovascular system and promote healthy eyes as well.

CUMIN has a strong, nutty, citrusy-peppery flavor. This spice is very high in iron, manganese, calcium, and magnesium.

CINNAMON reduces blood sugar and carb cravings.

MUSTARD SEED and CAYENNE PEPPER can boost your metabolism.

Last, but not least, TURMERIC is a powerful antioxidant.

The truly great thing about eating so simply is that you don't have to do a ton of preparation to start and keep eating well. The most real work you'll do is chopping your veggies into bite-size pieces, but if you're not presenting the food to Gordon Ramsay, the Michelin-star chef of *Hell's Kitchen* fame, you don't have to worry about perfect plating.

What You Need

Every cook needs a few tools. What's great about eating ketogenically is that you don't have to buy anything (other than food) or track down strange new devices. You just need good food and a few basic cooking tools.

A good cast iron pan. This can double as a pizza pan and roasting pan. Preferably 16-inch, but if you don't have a ton of kids, like me, you can go smaller.

A couple of good baking sheets for roasting or baking. Line them with foil for easy cleanup.

At least two knives. A paring knife and a chef's knife will come in handy. You can do anything with these two knives, as long as they're sharp.

Tongs, serving spoons, vegetable peelers, blenders, and mixers can be helpful, but they're not necessary. If you're a smoothie lover, a blender is going to be a priority.

Don't forget your **slow cooker**. If you have one, use it! You can place a whole keto meal in a slow cooker in the morning, and it will be done and waiting when you get home. Pulled pork, shredded beef, stews, and all sorts of dishes can be made in a slow cooker, and they will welcome you at the end of the day.

REMEMBER TO EXERCISE

Yes, you still have to exercise. But what's really great is that instead of killing yourself just to burn calories, on a keto diet, you're working to build strength and muscle mass instead of worrying about calorie loss.

Walk every day. Walk as much as possible. Park at the back of the parking lot, and walk to the store. Walk around the block on your lunch hour. As a mom, I spend a lot of time waiting for kids to finish their activities. I usually take this time—especially if the rest of my day is extra busy—to go for a walk. I walk 15 minutes out and then 15 minutes back.

Ride a bike. Riding a bike is a fantastic way to strengthen your body and get a cardio workout at the same time. Just holding onto the handlebars, steering, and dealing with bumps works your arms out more than you think—and of course the lower-body benefits are second to none. You don't have to be a serious biker either. Don't worry about getting tight pants and a yellow jersey. The great thing about bikes is you don't even have to go fast to get the benefits!

Lift things. One of the best ways to get lean is to lift things and do some work. You don't have to be a bodybuilder, but doing a kettlebell workout (I use a gallon of milk filled with water or sand) will give you a great workout—especially in the abs and arms. Lift buckets of water, and carry them out to your garden instead of using the hose. If you have back issues, look into other ways to add resistance to your exercise routine.

Run! Run like someone is chasing you. Then walk for a bit. Then sprint for a bit. A number of studies have shown that doing short bursts of intense exercise is actually better for your weight-loss efforts than long, sustained cardio. So, race to the telephone pole; then walk back. Or race up a hill; then walk down. Doing this for 20 or 30 minutes three or four times a week will bring on the sweat and lower the pounds. Always do what's comfortable for your health. Consult with a doctor if you'd like to add high-intensity running to your routine.

Play! You don't have to do a physical routine to get exercise. Do the dance game on your video game system. Play basketball or soccer. Walk on the beach and look for shells. Play Frisbee with your dog. Just have fun and add movement to your every day. You'll see a difference in how you look and feel.

PLAN AHEAD

Want to get a head start on the week ahead? Sit down and sort out your menu for the week. Once you know what you're going to eat and you have all your ingredients, you can spend around 30 minutes getting it sorted. Depending on how organized you want to be, you can either prep your vegetables and proteins and label them for each day or meal, or you can simply estimate about how many of each prepped vegetable you'll need and put them in zip bags or containers labeled with what's inside.

CUT ALL OF YOUR VEGETABLES AHEAD OF TIME. Most vegetables can be cut and kept fresh or frozen for the week ahead. Work from your hardest vegetables to cut, like squash or sweet potatoes, and move up to onions (which leave the most odor on the cutting board). Place each item in its own zip bag and label.

MARINATE MEATS. If you know you are eating taco salad or shredded beef or chicken for the beginning of the week, get them marinating now. Place your ingredients, meat, and liquid in a zip bag, and place it flat in the fridge. They'll practically be cooked by Tuesday or Wednesday when you're ready to use them!

FREEZE IT. If you have more than 30 minutes, make up a dish ahead of time and have it ready for after that Thursday night soccer game. You could easily roast a chicken ahead of time and pull half for chicken salad on Wednesday and eat the other half after you're done prepping for the week on Sunday night. (You *must* eat some of a chicken you just roasted).

ROAST A TURKEY. If you don't have a big family like me, make it a small one (¼ to ½ pound per person). But roast a turkey, and then those who aren't on a keto diet in the family can have turkey sandwiches or wraps all week—and you can have turkey to put on a salad, drape with dried eggs, and wrap up in lettuce for a keto-style wrap.

PART II

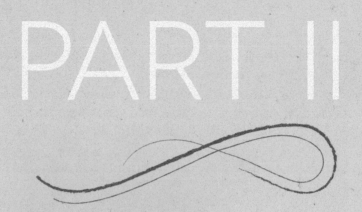

28-DAY
MEAL PLAN

THE RECIPES IN THIS MEAL PLAN are just guidelines, and there are many other delectable recipes in part 3. If you see a dish in the meal plan that does not appeal to you, simply swap it out for another recipe. The plan also incorporates leftovers to make your life easier.

Each day of the meal plan has suggestions for breakfast, lunch, and dinner with a perfect side dish. You get to pick at least 2 snacks from the handy weekly list, which offers 12 choices, and still keep your calories and net carbs in a range that supports weight loss. Eat your snacks, because 1,600 calories per day is too low for most people. Desserts are not included on the meal plan, but you can satisfy your sweet tooth with the choices in chapter 11, which are perfect for the keto lifestyle.

Each week has a shopping list that outlines all the ingredients you'll need for the week. Look in your fridge and pantry before going to the grocery store or farmers' market, and check off any items you already have on hand. Be sure to add the ingredients for the snacks you choose to your shopping list.

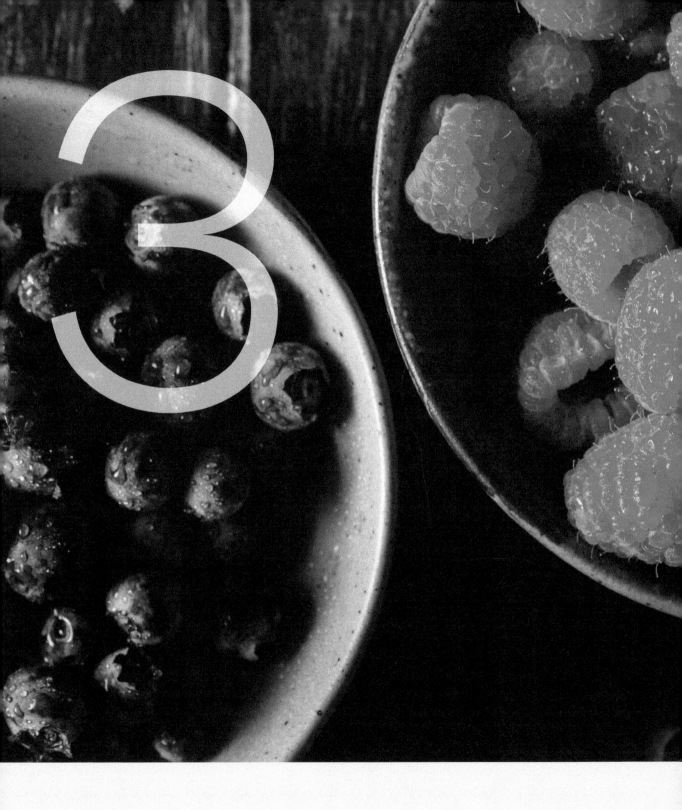

THE PLAN

The nitty-gritty. The nuts and bolts. This is the plan—in all its wonderful detail—that will keep you on track for the first four weeks of your keto journey. Everything you need is laid out in the following chapter, from what to eat for breakfast to how many slices of bacon you'll need for the week. Yes, *need*. Each day's macronutrient break down is listed, along with the net carbs for easy tracking. There are lists of snacks in case hunger strikes between meals, and bit of encouragement at the beginning of each week to help you stay the course. Four weeks from now, you'll be able to make your own plan for moving forward.

WEEK ONE

This is the first week in your journey to eating a keto diet, and you might experience some significant changes in your routine and body as the week progresses. If you are not a culinary whiz or do not habitually cook your meals, the time spent shopping and creating the meals might be overwhelming. Ideally, schedule a slow week to help your body adjust to the new diet.

The extent of your withdrawal symptoms will depend on the amount of carbs in your current diet, the amount of exercise you do, and how much glucose is stored in your body when you start the week. Most people hit the carb withdrawal wall on day three or four. The symptoms include hunger, muscle aches, headache, fatigue, mental fogginess, and dizziness. Make sure you hydrate and eat adequate salt to keep your sodium levels up. You should feel better by the end of the week and will probably be in ketosis as you start week two.

WEEK ONE MENU

	BREAKFAST	LUNCH	DINNER
MONDAY 70% fat 5% carbs 25% protein 16g net carbs	Creamy Cinnamon Breakfast Pudding	Ground Beef Taco Salad	Grilled Venison Loin with Dijon Cream Sauce Sesame-Roasted Broccoli
TUESDAY 71% fat 7% carbs 22% protein 17g net carbs	Simple Scrambled Eggs	Walnut-Fennel Salad with Sherry Vinaigrette	Ham-Stuffed Pork Chops Broccoli-Cauliflower Casserole
WEDNESDAY 72% fat 8% carbs 20% protein 15g net carbs	Buttery Coconut Bread	Jalapeño Frittata	Chicken Milanese Brussels Sprouts with Hazelnuts
THURSDAY 70% fat 10% carbs 20% protein 16g net carbs	Buttery Coconut Bread	Asian Shrimp Salad	Sole Meunière Roasted Asparagus with Goat Cheese
FRIDAY 70% fat 7% carbs 23% protein 15g net carbs	Fluffy Baked Omelet with Pancetta and Swiss Cheese	Watercress-Spinach Soup	Caprese Balsamic Chicken Creamed Spinach
SATURDAY 70% fat 8% carbs 22% protein 16g net carbs	Corned Beef Breakfast Hash	Chicken Caesar Salad	Sea Scallops with Bacon Cream Sauce Cauliflower "Rice"
SUNDAY 70% fat 10% carbs 20% protein 16g net carbs	Spanakopita Omelet	Lemon Smoothie	Rich Sausage Casserole Walnut-Fennel Salad with Sherry Vinaigrette

SNACKS (CHOOSE ONE OR TWO EACH DAY)

Beef Jerky

Cheesy Shrimp Spread

Cold Cuts and Cheese Roll-Ups

Creamy Kale Smoothie

Hard-boiled Egg

Lemon Smoothie

Nuts (Walnuts, Pecans, Macadamia)

Cheesecake Smoothie

Olives Stuffed with Feta Cheese

Peanut Butter Cookies

Simple Cheesy Yogurt

String Cheese

WEEK ONE SHOPPING LIST

Meat, Poultry, Seafood

Bacon (15 slices)

Black forest ham (4 slices)

Chicken breasts (5, 8-ounce)

Corned beef (8 ounces)

Ground beef, 25% fat (½ pound)

Lean ham (¼ pound)

Pancetta (4 ounces)

Pork chops, center cut (4, 4-ounce)

Pork sausage meat (½ pound)

Sea scallops (1 pound)

Shrimp (16–20 count, ½ pound)

Sole fillets (4, 4-ounce)

Turkey bacon (8 slices)

Venison loin (1 pound)

Dairy

Butter (2½ cups)

Cheese, Cheddar, shredded (2¼ cups)

Cheese, cottage (16 ounces)

Cheese, cream (14 ounces)

Cheese, feta (1 cup)

Cheese, goat (10 ounces)

Cheese, mozzarella, shredded (1 cup)

Cheese, Parmesan (6 ounces)

Cheese, Swiss (4 slices)

Cheese, Swiss, shredded (1 cup)

Eggs (4 dozen)

Heavy (whipping) cream (5 cups)

Produce

Arugula (4 ounces)

Asparagus (2 pounds, about 30 spears)

Avocado (2)

Basil, fresh (1 bunch)

Broccoli (3½ pounds, or 4 heads)

Brussels sprouts (¾ pound)

Cauliflower (3 heads)

Chives, fresh (1 bunch)

Cilantro, fresh (1 bunch)

Fennel (1 head)

Fresh oregano (1 bunch)

Garlic (16 cloves, or 8½ teaspoons minced)

Green bell pepper (1)

Jalapeño pepper (4)

Lemon (6)

Lime (1)

Mint, fresh (1 bunch)

Oregano, fresh (1 bunch)

Parsley, fresh (1 bunch)

Red bell pepper (1)

Romaine lettuce (4 heads)

Rosemary, fresh (1 bunch)

Scallions (4)

Shallots (2)

Snow peas (2 ounces)

Spaghetti squash (1)

Spinach (22 ounces)

Sweet onion (1)

Tarragon, fresh (1 bunch)

Thyme, fresh (2 bunches)

Tomato (2)

Watercress (2 bunches)

White mushrooms (½ pound)

WEEK TWO

Congratulations on finishing week one of the keto lifestyle! You have committed to making a change and are following through on the plan. You are probably in ketosis by the beginning of week two, especially if you exercise moderately and stick to the meal plan. You might have even lost some weight and may be noticing that your appetite has diminished without the constant intake of carbs.

You should be over any carb withdrawal symptoms and starting to get used to the routine of cooking and eating foods high in fat. Take a look at the meal plan, and pinpoint any days that you might be extra busy so you can adjust the plan to suit your time constraints. For example, you can double up on a recipe so that you have leftovers for the next evening. Just adjust the shopping list to reflect the change.

Keep an eye on your protein levels so that they don't creep up, because too much protein will prevent ketosis. The recipes in your meal plan will be balanced to prevent any overage. Make sure you keep hydrating because your body will not retain water the same way when you are in a state of ketosis.

WEEK TWO MENU

	BREAKFAST	LUNCH	DINNER
MONDAY 72% fat 7% carbs 21% protein 19g net carbs	Creamy Cinnamon Breakfast Pudding	Cobb Salad	Rib Eye Steaks with Garlic-Thyme Butter Buttery Mashed Cauliflower
TUESDAY 70% fat 9% carbs 21% protein 20g net carbs	Applesauce Yogurt Muffins	Peanut-Chicken Soup	Golden Fried Fish Stuffed Portobello Mushrooms
WEDNESDAY 70% fat 6% carbs 24% protein 18g net carbs	Fluffy Baked Omelet with Pancetta and Swiss Cheese	Asian Shrimp Salad	Swedish Meatballs Zucchini Fritters
THURSDAY 72% fat 6% carbs 22% protein 18g net carbs	Spiced Cream Cheese Pancakes Cinnamon-Caramel Sauce	Seafood Chowder	Coconut Chicken Cauliflower "Rice"
FRIDAY 70% fat 8% carbs 22% protein 15g net carbs	Breakfast "Sandwich"	Cucumber Green Smoothie	Grilled Venison Loin with Dijon Cream Sauce Spinach Soufflé
SATURDAY 70% fat 8% carbs 22% protein 17g net carbs	Vanilla Belgian Waffles	Chicken Caesar Salad	Barbecued Shrimp with Avocado Salsa Coconut-Zucchini Noodles
SUNDAY 72% fat 8% carbs 20% protein 17% net carbs	Egg Breakfast Muffins	Jalapeño-Chicken Soup	Casserole au Gratin

SNACKS (CHOOSE ONE OR TWO EACH DAY)

Cheesecake Smoothie	Coconut Tzatziki	Beef Jerky
Chocolate-Mint Smoothie	Chocolate Fudge	Avocado Slices
Peanut Butter Smoothie	Hard-boiled Egg	Broccoli, Cauliflower, or Celery with Ranch Dip
Goat Cheese Nuggets	Celery with Peanut Butter	
	Nuts (Walnuts, Pecans, Macadamia)	

WEEK TWO SHOPPING LIST

Meat, Poultry, and Seafood

Bacon (20 slices)

Chicken breasts, boneless and skinless (4, 8-ounce)

Chicken thighs, boneless and skinless (½ pound)

Ground beef (¾ pound)

Ground pork (¾ pound)

Haddock fillets (1 pound)

Lean ham (¾ pound)

Lobster meat, cooked (2 cups)

Pancetta (4 ounces)

Peameal bacon (4 slices)

Rib eye steaks (4, 6-ounce)

Shrimp, 16–20 count (1¾ pound)

Venison loin (1 pound)

Dairy

Butter (3½ cups)

Cheese, aged Cheddar (16 ounces)

Cheese, blue (2 ounces)

Cheese, cottage (32 ounces)

Cheese, cream (30 ounces)

Cheese, goat (1 ounce)

Cheese, Jack, shredded (2½ cups)

Cheese, mozzarella, shredded (¼ cup)

Cheese, Parmesan (8 ounces)

Cheese, Swiss, shredded (1 cup)

Eggs (5 dozen)

Greek yogurt (1¼ cup)

Heavy (whipping) cream (7 cups)

Sour cream (8 ounces)

Produce

Asparagus (1 bunch)

Avocados (2)

Basil, fresh (1 bunch)

Carrot (1)

Cauliflower (4 heads)

Celery stalks (3)

Chives (1 bunch)

Cilantro, fresh (1 bunch)

English cucumber (1)

Garlic (22 cloves, or 11 teaspoons minced)

Jalapeño peppers (7)

Kale (1 bunch)

Leek (½)

Lemons (3)

Limes (4)

Mixed mushrooms (4 cups)

Parsley, fresh (1 bunch)

Portobello mushrooms (4)

Red bell pepper (2)

Romaine lettuce (3 heads)

Rosemary, fresh (1 bunch)

Scallions (3)

Snow peas (2 ounces)

Spinach (10 ounces)

Sweet onion (4)

Tahini (1 tablespoon)

Thyme, fresh (1 bunch)

Tomatoes, cherry (1 pint)

Tomatoes, sun-dried, packed in oil (6 tomatoes)

Zucchini (3 pounds)

WEEK THREE

You are now officially just over halfway to completing your first 28 days of eating a keto diet. You should be seeing and feeling some results from all your hard work, so it is important to stick with the plan. You might find yourself having some sugar cravings this week, so swap out one of the snack options for dessert, such as Chocolate Parfaits (page 197) or Lemon Cheesecake (page 206).

You should have plenty of energy but might not be up to your usual workout levels yet. This is normal, so if you are not up to a full workout, take a brisk walk instead or a swim in the local pool. It is important to keep exercising, but don't overdo it if you feel your body is not performing.

After two weeks on the meal plan, you should have some new favorite dishes you might want to use instead of the suggested meals. Take a look at the recipe you want to use, and compare it to the meal plan recommendation to ensure the fat, carb, and protein percentages are similar.

WEEK THREE MENU

	BREAKFAST	LUNCH	DINNER
MONDAY 71% fat 9% carbs 20% protein 16g net carbs	Buttery Coconut Bread	Ground Beef Taco Salad	Herb-Infused Chicken Broccoli-Cauliflower Casserole
TUESDAY 71% fat 8% carbs 21% protein 18g net carbs	Buttery Coconut Bread	Fiesta Lime Chicken Chowder	Spicy Crab Cakes Spinach Soufflé
WEDNESDAY 73% fat 5% carbs 22% protein 15g net carbs	Fluffy Baked Omelet with Pancetta and Swiss Cheese	Walnut-Fennel Salad with Sherry Vinaigrette	Pan-Grilled Lamb Chops with Herb Pesto Whole Roasted Cauliflower
THURSDAY 71% fat 7% carbs 22% protein 17g net carbs	Chia Almond "Oatmeal"	Chicken Caesar Salad	Sole Meunière Twice-Baked Spaghetti Squash
FRIDAY 70% fat 7% carbs 23% protein 20g net carbs	Jalapeño Frittata	Country Pork and "Rice" Soup	Italian Meatballs Roasted Asparagus with Goat Cheese
SATURDAY 70% fat 10% carbs 20% protein 17g net carbs	Spiced Cream Cheese Pancakes Pastry Cream	Cobb Salad	Chicken Milanese Cauliflower "Rice"
SUNDAY 70% fat 6% carbs 24% protein 15g net carbs	Spanakopita Omelet	Chicken Salad–Stuffed Avocados	Bacon-Wrapped Beef Tenderloin Creamed Spinach

SNACKS (CHOOSE ONE OR TWO EACH DAY)

Chocolate-Mint Smoothie

Avocado-Lime Smoothie

Peanut Butter Smoothie

Guacamole

Nut Crackers

Cold Cuts and Cheese Roll-Ups

Olives Stuffed with Feta Cheese

Bacon Slices

Nuts (Walnuts, Pecans, Macadamia)

Broccoli, Cauliflower, or Celery with Ranch Dip

Sardines

WEEK THREE SHOPPING LIST

Meat, Poultry, and Seafood

Bacon (27 slices)

Beef tenderloin steaks (4, 4-ounce)

Chicken breasts, skin on (4, 8-ounce)

Chicken thighs, bone in (4, 7-ounce)

Chicken thighs, boneless skinless (½ pound)

Country pork ribs, boneless (1 pound)

Crab (1 pound)

Ground beef, 25% fat (1¼ pounds)

Lamb chops (4, 4-ounce)

Lean ham (¼ pound)

Pancetta (6 ounces)

Sole fillets (4, 4-ounce)

Dairy

Butter (2¼ cups)

Cheese, aged Cheddar (36 ounces)

Cheese, blue (2 ounces)

Cheese, cottage (16 ounces)

Cheese, cream (28 ounces)

Cheese, feta (1 cup)

Cheese, goat (7 ounces)

Cheese, Parmesan (5 ounces)

Cheese, Swiss, shredded (1 cup)

Eggs (5 dozen)

Produce

Arugula (4 ounces)

Asparagus (2 pounds, or about 30 spears)

Avocados (4)

Basil, fresh (1 bunch)

Blueberries, dried

Broccoli (1 pound, or 1 head)

Cauliflower (3 heads)

Chives, fresh (1 bunch)

Cilantro, fresh (1 bunch)

Cranberries, dried

Dill, fresh (1 bunch)

Fennel (1 head)

Garlic (27 cloves, or 13½ teaspoons minced)

Green bell pepper (1)

Jalapeño peppers (4)

Lemons (7)

Lime (1)

Mint, fresh (1 bunch)

Oregano, fresh (1 bunch)

Parsley, fresh (1 bunch)

Red bell pepper (1)

Red onion (1)

Romaine lettuce (3 heads)

Rosemary, fresh (1 bunch)

Scallions (4)

Shallots (3)

Spaghetti squash (1)

Spinach (26 ounces)

Sweet onions (2)

Tarragon, fresh (1 bunch)

Thyme, fresh (1 bunch)

Tomato (1)

Tomatoes, cherry (1 pint)

White mushrooms (½ pound)

Wine, dry white

WEEK FOUR

How do you feel?

You are officially in the home stretch of the 28-day keto diet plan, so pat yourself on the back for everything you have achieved so far. In the fourth week of the plan, you will have lost weight. The amount of weight depends on your physical state at the beginning of this journey, your activity level, and how well you have kept to the diet.

You have probably noticed increased energy levels, reduced food cravings, and improved digestive health along with the lower number on the scale. Reaching for a ripe avocado or munching on crisp, salty bacon as a snack should seem natural and satisfying. If you have not tried other recipes in this book yet, after this week, you can start compiling your own meal plan and discovering many more delicious meal choices.

It takes about 21 days to change a habit and develop new ones, so this last week will solidify your new low-carb, high-fat lifestyle.

WEEK FOUR MENU

	BREAKFAST	LUNCH	DINNER
MONDAY 70% fat 7% carbs 23% protein 17g net carbs	Cucumber Green Smoothie	Country Pork and "Rice" Soup	Caprese Balsamic Chicken Broccoli-Cauliflower Casserole
TUESDAY 73% fat 6% carbs 21% protein 15g net carbs	Spanakopita Omelet	Walnut-Fennel Salad with Sherry Vinaigrette	Grilled Venison Loin with Dijon Cream Sauce Creamed Spinach
WEDNESDAY 70% fat 10% carbs 20% protein 20g net carbs	Chia Almond "Oatmeal"	Peanut-Chicken Soup	Ham-Stuffed Pork Chops Stuffed Portobello Mushrooms
THURSDAY 71% fat 6% carbs 23% protein 17g net carbs	Creamy Cinnamon Breakfast Pudding	Jalapeño Frittata	Baked Halibut with Herb Sauce Twice-Baked Spaghetti Squash
FRIDAY 70% fat 8% carbs 22% protein 18g net carbs	Skillet-Baked Eggs with Yogurt and Spinach	Seafood Chowder	Beef Stroganoff Buttery Mashed Cauliflower
SATURDAY 73% fat 7% carbs 20% protein 17g net carbs	"Cornbread" Muffins Simple Cheesy Yogurt	Sirloin Steak Salad with Goat Cheese and Pecans	Casserole au Gratin
SUNDAY 71% fat 9% carbs 20% protein 16g net carbs	Vanilla Belgian Waffles Cinnamon-Caramel Sauce	Fiesta Lime Chicken Chowder	Brown Butter–Lime Tilapia Coconut-Zucchini Noodles

SNACKS (CHOOSE ONE OR TWO EACH DAY)

Cheesecake Smoothie	Parmesan Crisps	Cold Cuts and Cheese Roll-Ups
Chocolate-Mint Smoothie	Toasty Granola Bars	Beef Jerky
Vanilla Bean Smoothie	Celery with Cream Cheese	Avocado Slices
Orange Cream Ice Pops	Hard-boiled Egg	Bacon Slices

WEEK FOUR SHOPPING LIST

Meats, Poultry, and Seafood

Black forest ham (4 slices)

Chicken breasts, boneless and skinless (3, 6-ounce)

Chicken thighs, boneless and skinless (½ pound)

Country pork ribs, boneless (1 pound)

Halibut fillet (4, 5-ounce)

Lean ham (1 pound)

Lobster meat (2 cups)

Pancetta (6 slices)

Pork chops, center cut (4, 4-ounce)

Shrimp (¼ pound)

Tilapia fillets (4, 4-ounce)

Top sirloin steak (1¼ pound)

Venison loin (1 pound)

Dairy

Butter (3¼ cup)

Cheese, Cheddar, shredded (1¼ cups)

Cheese, cottage (16 ounces)

Cheese, cream (38 ounces)

Cheese, feta (1 cup)

Cheese, goat (9 ounces)

Cheese, mozzarella, shredded (1¼ cup)

Cheese, Parmesan (2 ounces)

Cheese, Swiss (4 slices)

Eggs (4 dozen)

Sour cream (6 ounces)

Produce

Arugula (4 ounces)

Asparagus (1 pound)

Avocado (1)

Broccoli (1 head)

Cauliflower (4 heads)

Celery stalks (2)

Chives, fresh (1 bunch)

Cilantro (1 bunch)

Dill, fresh (1 bunch)

English cucumber (1)

Fennel (1 head)

Garlic (35 cloves, or 17½ teaspoons minced)

Jalapeño peppers (4)

Kale (1 cup)

Leek (1)

Lemons (2)

Lime (1)

Mint, fresh (1 bunch)

Oregano, fresh (1 bunch)

Parsley, fresh (1 bunch)

Portobello mushrooms (4)

Romaine (1 head)

Rosemary, fresh (1 bunch)

Scallion (1)

Shallots (2)

Spaghetti squash (1)

Spinach (26 ounces)

Sweet onion (4)

Thyme, fresh (1 bunch)

Tomato (3)

White mushrooms (¾ pound)

Zucchini (3)

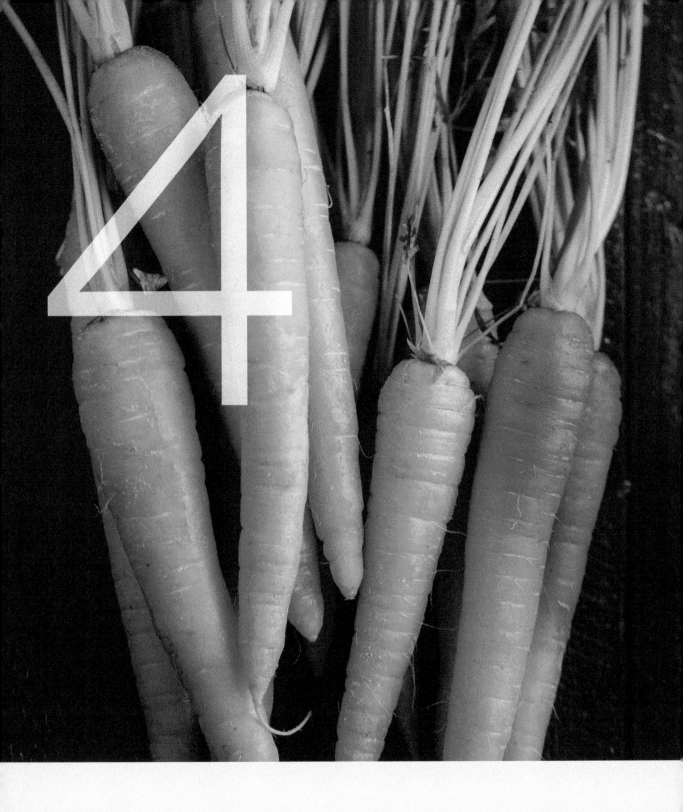

BEYOND YOUR FIRST 28 DAYS

At first, it might seem that maintaining a ketogenic lifestyle will be difficult; I can say from experience, it doesn't have to be hard. Will you crave bread once in a while? Sure. Will you want to eat cake? Maybe. The great thing about eating a low- to no-carb diet is that after a while, you simply don't want carbs anymore. When you're tempted occasionally and cave (which I do), it's not nearly as satisfying as you think it's going to be. In fact, I've found giving in to be a little disappointing and not worth it over all. However, there will be bumpy patches and times when you're just going to say, "Forget it. I'm eating this ramen because I want to, and no stupid diet can tell me otherwise." That's okay. Eat the ramen. Denying yourself something you think you want only makes you resent the diet, and that's not the point.

MAINTAINING A KETO LIFESTYLE

In that vein, here are a few tips to help you on the path to maintaining your new lifestyle:

Have a cheat day (after the first 28). One cheat day per week is something to look forward to. After years of doing this, I really don't "need" a cheat day anymore. Your body will start to slow down its rate of weight loss when it's on any kind of routine. A cheat day can actually boost your metabolism by throwing something "new" at your body. Technically you'll be out of ketosis, but you don't want to be in ketosis all the time anyway. You want to mix it up a bit after the first month or so. It's important to keep your metabolism guessing a bit—that's what keeps it working.

Join an online support group or discussion forum. There are a number of places online, including Facebook groups, completely devoted to folks who are eating ketogenically. All of them are devoted to learning more about it. Join up with them! When you're having a hard, carb-flu day, you can talk to others who've been there and get their advice or just chat.

Travel prepared. When you're traveling, and this includes commuting or dropping kids off at all kinds of activities, have snacks with you that will keep you satisfied and keep you from going through the drive-through. Keep macadamias on hand or beef jerky. And if you do go through the drive-through, skip the fries and eat the burger or chicken with lettuce instead of a bun.

Eat what you like. Do this especially when you're having a hard day. It is way better to go ahead and make yourself a BLT—no bread, of course—than it is to think you have to eat salmon every night, especially if you don't like salmon. Choose the foods that really appeal to you (I like pulled pork and would eat it almost every night), and stick to those.

Go to the grocery store instead of the convenience store or a restaurant when you're in a different town. I have found all kinds of great low-carb snack options when I choose the grocery store instead of the convenience store. One night I picked out prosciutto and mozzarella cheese rolls in a little deli pack. Perfect! Avocados are also great travel food—just slice down the middle, take out the pit and eat them with a spoon, right out of their own handy package.

Use your slow cooker! A slow cooker is one of the best tools a keto dieter can have. Put a pork roast in it in the morning, and then shred it for two or three meals later on. Lettuce wraps are great with a taco-style pulled pork dish, or try "enchiladas" wrapped in large kale leaves instead of tortillas. These are so many delicious ways to use pork cooked slow and pulled. I like pulled pork; can you tell?

Freeze meals ahead of time. One of the best ways to save money and carbs is to make up a few meals on Sunday and freeze them for the rest of the week. Instead of being tempted by hunger when you come home and ordering a pizza, you'll have a dinner plan all set. Just pull out whatever you made for that day, pop it in the oven, and in the same amount of time it would have taken the delivery guy to get there, your dinner is done.

Use your leftovers. Leftovers make your lunch the next day so simple, and since you cooked it, you know just what's in it. Bring leftovers to work or school, or transform them into something a little different—add last night's stir-fry to an omelet, for example.

Make your snacks protein or fat rich! Hard-boiled eggs, cheese, and jerky are all great snacks. When you find yourself craving sweets, go for some fat. Fry up some cheese in coconut oil, put bacon fat on fried veggies, or eat kelp or kale chips to get through a snacky time.

KEEPING UP YOUR EXERCISE ROUTINE

If you didn't exercise much before, now is a good time to start. But you can certainly wait until the "carb flu" is over. While it may seem overwhelming to start a new diet and a new workout routine, truth be told, it may be easier to start them both at the same time. In fact, your new commitment to your health might be just the impetus you need to get going!

Now, before you run out the door and down the block, think about your routine and the kind of exercise you want to do. Many people take on CrossFit-style (weight lifting, high intensity, low cardio) exercises when they start a ketogenic routine. Weights and resistance work are a good place to begin, as long as you start out slowly. Others are more comfortable with cardio-style exercises or group classes. It really doesn't matter what type of exercise you pick in the beginning; it's just important that you get your body moving. It's not about burning calories on a ketogenic diet; it's about building strength and stamina.

Here are a few tips to help you on the path to maintaining the exercise component of your keto lifestyle:

Pick a time of day that works for you. Don't go telling yourself you're going to get up at 5 a.m. and run three miles if you're really not going to do it. I used to do this, and then I berated myself for not getting up on time or being too sleepy. Now I know I'm going to drink coffee and work until 9 a.m., and then I'll take a break to walk or run the dogs.

Get into a routine. I walk every day at 9 a.m., and then I walk or bike ride every afternoon around 4 p.m. That's what works best for me and my schedule. If I don't do it, or I'm not home at those times, I feel weird.

Exercise wherever you are. Just because you aren't in a gym or at home doesn't mean you can't exercise. Go shoot hoops at the corner basket while your kids are at practice. Take a walk while your kid is at dance class. Ride your bike home from work. Jumping jacks can be done anywhere. Fit it in, and you'll get fit.

Move. Wherever you are and whatever you're doing, move around. Cooking dinner? Do a few squats while waiting for the water to boil. In line at the bank? Do a few toe raises. Walking up the stairs? Run them. The more you move, the better you'll feel.

Sleep. Don't neglect your sleep. The best way to screw up a workout routine is to not sleep. Sleep. Take a nap. Let your body—and your hormones—rest. It's one of the best things you can do for your weight-loss plan.

TEMPTED BY OLD WAYS?

Take heart. It happens to all of us, and it's okay. Here's some help in managing old temptations:

Give yourself permission to eat. If grandma's made a pie, and you want a piece of it, have one. Being healthy in our food choices means we can give ourselves permission to eat but not overeat. Indulge—in small doses.

Be kind to yourself. You may eat that piece of fudge or whatever while on the boardwalk at the beach. Maybe it puts you to 50 or 80 carbs for the day. But think about how good that is in comparison to where you once were. It's okay. Start clean on the next day.

Follow the 80/20 principle. If you eat extremely well 80 percent of your week, that leftover 20 percent is not going to hurt you. Waiting until after your initial 28 days to implement this principle is best.

Drink water. Want that sweet snack? Drink a glass of water first. Want to eat a piece of pizza? Drink a glass of water. Put something in it like lemon or lime. Drink fizzy water. Drink unsweetened iced tea. Chances are, a belly full of liquid will help you pass over that big cookie. Walk on. Have a drink.

Smell it. I've been able to satisfy my craving for cookies, bread, and all kinds of things by allowing myself to smell them and then just walking on by, glass of water in hand. It sounds silly, but if taste is mostly about smell, I can see why this works.

MAKE YOUR OWN MEAL PLAN

Sit down and write a list of 10 or 20 of your favorite dinners. Invite your family or friends to help you with this activity. Then go through those ingredients and figure out how to make your plan keto. You know the drill by now. Consult "Pantry Essentials" and "The Keto Spice Rack" in chapter 2 for ideas, and browse through the shopping lists in chapter 3 for further inspiration. After that, you'll be ready to plan your adapted meals for the week. You can concentrate on breakfasts, lunches, or dinners. Perhaps you'd like to experiment with making all three meals every other day. Remember "Maintaining a Keto Lifestyle" at the beginning of this chapter? Well, getting creative with your own meal planning is another way to keep up all your good work!

PART III

RECIPES

HERE WE ARE—THE GOOD STUFF. These recipes
will quickly become your new comfort foods, and with good reason.
Sumptuous dishes will delight you from breakfast to dessert; you might
even forget that you're following a plan! The recipes included in the
following chapters go well beyond those listed in the plan so that you'll
never lack for variety. You might be shocked to discover how easy
and satisfying it is to make your own pantry staples, discover a new
favorite breakfast, or find an entrée to replace your go-to dinner party
recipe. Most of all, enjoy!

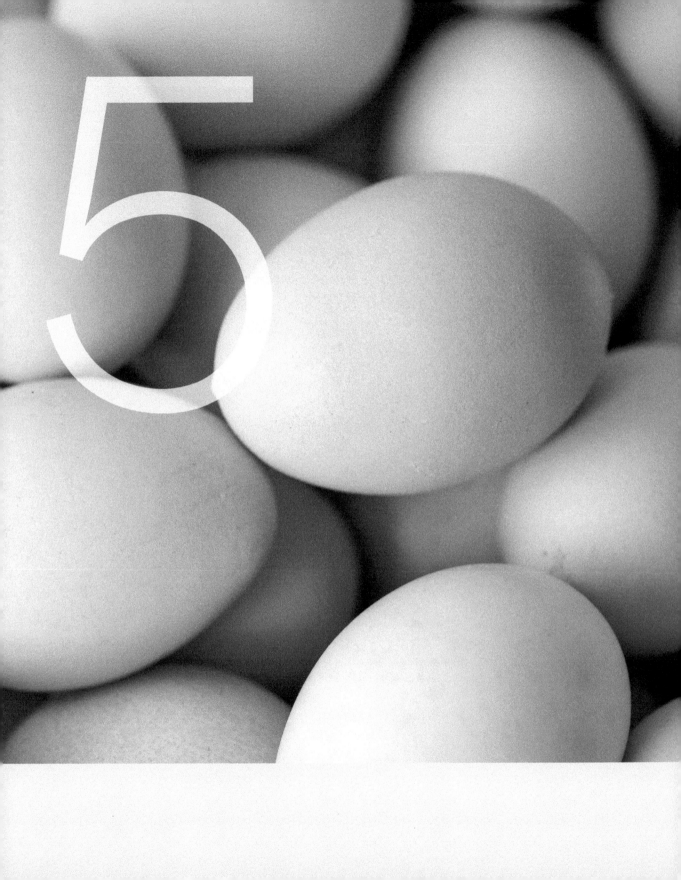

BREAKFAST

Creamy Cinnamon Breakfast Pudding

SERVES 4 / PREP TIME: 2 MINUTES / COOK TIME: 11 MINUTES

2 cups cottage cheese

1 cup heavy (whipping) cream

4 large eggs

2 tablespoons flaxseed meal

4 (7g) stevia packets

½ teaspoon ground cinnamon

¼ teaspoon ground nutmeg

¼ cup butter, for topping

IN MENU FOR WEEKS:

A CLOSER LOOK: *A natural sweetener extracted from plants, stevia is grown mostly in Brazil and Paraguay. This popular sugar substitute is over 200 times sweeter than granulated sugar, so add it sparingly and test the sweetness of your food. You can find stevia in both liquid and granulated forms.*

Under 30 Minutes • One Pot • Make Ahead *A filling, hot pudding can be exactly what you need to start the day off right. The texture of the cooked eggs, cottage cheese, and flaxseed will remind you of cream of wheat, and the flavor is reminiscent of warm gingerbread. You might want to stir the golden melted butter topping into the pudding, or you might scoop it all up in the first few spoonfuls.*

1. In a medium saucepan over medium-high heat, whisk the cottage cheese, heavy cream, and eggs to combine.

2. Cook the cheese mixture, stirring occasionally, until the mixture starts to boil, about 5 minutes.

3. Reduce the heat and simmer until the eggs are cooked through, about 4 minutes.

4. Remove the saucepan from the heat, and stir in the flaxseed meal, stevia, cinnamon, and nutmeg.

5. Divide the pudding evenly among 4 bowls, and top each with 1 tablespoon of butter. Serve immediately.

PER SERVING: CALORIES: 401 / FAT: 35G / TOTAL CARBS: 7G
FIBER: 1G / NET CARBS: 6G / SUGAR: 1G / PROTEIN: 18G

Fat 75% / Carbs 7% / Protein 18%   Ratio: 2:1

Vanilla Belgian Waffles

SERVES 4 / PREP TIME: 10 MINUTES, PLUS 15 MINUTES TO REST / COOK TIME: 20 MINUTES

Under 30 Minutes *You might think that waffles need to be drenched in syrup to be delicious; however, authentic Belgian waffles are served plain, dusted with a little confectioners' sugar, or topped with sliced strawberries and whipped cream. These waffles do not need a pile of toppings to enhance their crispy, golden goodness. You will need a waffle maker to create this dish as it is meant to be, but you can also use the batter in a skillet to make fluffy pancakes.*

1. In a large bowl, whisk the eggs until they are very frothy, about 3 minutes.

2. Whisk in the coconut milk, butter, and vanilla until blended.

3. Whisk the coconut flour, baking soda, and salt into the egg mixture until the batter is smooth and thick, about 1 minute.

4. Let the batter rest for 15 minutes so the coconut flour can thicken it.

5. Heat up the waffle maker, and make the waffles according to the manufacturer's directions.

6. Divide the waffles evenly among 4 plates, and serve.

8 large eggs, at room temperature

½ cup canned coconut milk

¼ cup butter, melted

½ teaspoon pure vanilla extract

½ cup coconut flour

¼ teaspoon baking soda

¼ teaspoon sea salt

IN MENU FOR WEEKS:

PER SERVING: CALORIES: 384 / FAT: 31G / TOTAL CARBS: 11G
FIBER: 7G / NET CARBS: 4G / SUGAR: 3G / PROTEIN: 16G

Fat 73% / Carbs 10% / Protein 17%   Ratio: 2:1

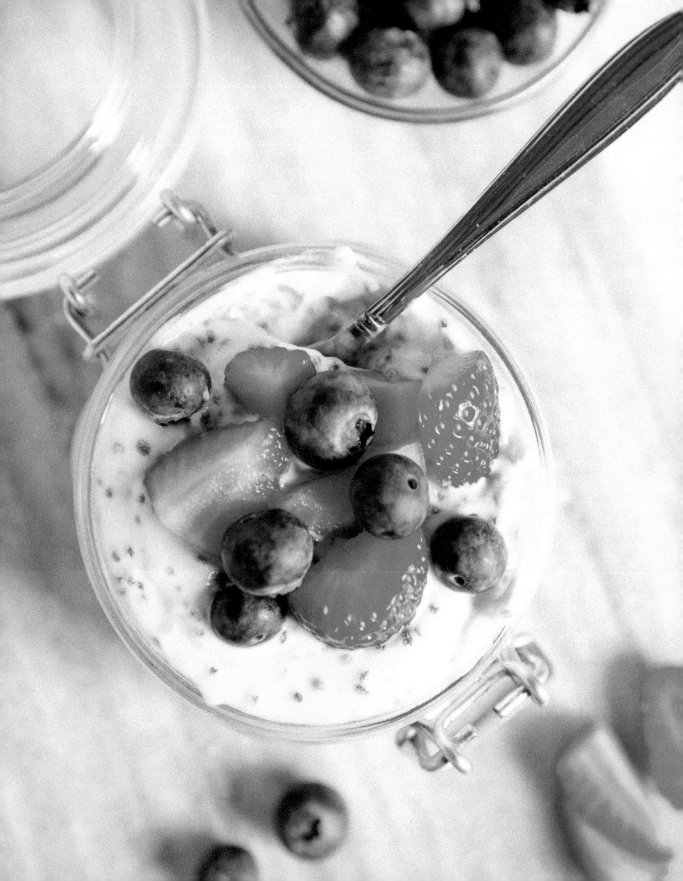

Chia Almond "Oatmeal"

SERVES 4 / PREP TIME: 10 MINUTES, PLUS 30 MINUTES TO COOL AND OVERNIGHT TO SOAK / COOK TIME: 5 MINUTES

One Pot • Make Ahead *Coconut plays a key role in the flavor and texture of this dish, both as milk and the shredded meat. If you want exceptional taste, you can crack a coconut yourself and grate or shred fresh coconut. First you drain out the liquid in the middle by piercing the soft "eye" with a sharp, thin tool, and then use the blunt side of a chef's knife to whack all the way around the circumference of the coconut until it cracks open. If it's your first time cracking a coconut, check out how-to videos on YouTube.*

1. Pour the water and coconut milk into a medium saucepan, and use a paring knife to scrape the vanilla seeds out of the pod into the liquid. Add the bean pod.

2. Place the saucepan over medium heat, and bring the liquid to a simmer, about 5 minutes.

3. Remove the pan from the heat, and set aside to cool for 30 minutes.

4. Remove and discard the vanilla bean.

5. In a medium bowl, stir to mix the chia seeds, coconut, and almonds.

6. Pour the cooled coconut milk liquid over the chia seed mixture, and stir to blend.

7. Place the "oatmeal" in the fridge overnight, covered, to allow the chia seeds to soak up all the liquid.

8. Stir in the stevia, divide the "oatmeal" evenly among 4 bowls, and serve topped with berries.

2 cups water

¾ cup coconut milk

1 vanilla bean, halved

½ cup chia seeds

¼ cup shredded unsweetened coconut

¼ cup slivered almonds

3 (7g) stevia packets

¼ cup mixed berries

IN MENU FOR WEEK:

3

A CLOSER LOOK: *Chia seeds come from a flowering member of the mint family, and these humble seeds are packed with omega-3 fatty acids, protein, calcium, and phosphorus. Chia seeds can help stabilize blood sugar and decrease the risk of insulin resistance and heart disease.*

PER SERVING: CALORIES: 219 / FAT: 18G / TOTAL CARBS: 16G
FIBER: 9G / NET CARBS: 7G / SUGAR: 3G / PROTEIN: 9G

Fat 74% / Carbs 16% / Protein 10%   Ratio: 3:1

Spiced Cream Cheese Pancakes

SERVES 4 / PREP TIME: 15 MINUTES / COOK TIME: 10 MINUTES

8 ounces cream cheese, softened

6 large eggs

3 (7g) stevia packets

¾ cup almond flour

1 teaspoon ground cinnamon

¼ teaspoon ground nutmeg

Pinch ground allspice

¼ cup butter, plus more for serving

IN MENU FOR WEEKS:

Under 30 Minutes *Cream cheese–based pancakes appear flatter than traditional pancakes, more crêpe-like than fluffy. The taste is rich and slightly tangy from the cheese, so syrup topping is not necessary to give this breakfast flavor. Try a few sweet raspberries, a dollop of heavy whipped cream, or Cinnamon-Caramel Sauce (page 223) to top off your short stack.*

1. In a blender, pulse the cream cheese, eggs, stevia, almond flour, cinnamon, nutmeg, and allspice until the mixture is very smooth.

2. In a large skillet on medium-high heat, heat 1 tablespoon of butter.

3. When the butter is sizzling, pour batter for 4 pancakes, about ¼ cup each, into the skillet.

4. Cook until the underside is golden, and flip the pancakes over, about 2 minutes.

5. Cook until the second side is golden, about 2 minutes.

6. Transfer the pancakes to plates, and repeat the process with 1 tablespoon of butter and the remaining batter.

7. Serve the pancakes topped with butter.

PER SERVING (2 PANCAKES): CALORIES: 410 / FAT: 33G
TOTAL CARBS: 9G / FIBER: 3G / NET CARBS: 6G
SUGAR: 3G / PROTEIN: 17G

Fat 73% / Carbs 10% / Protein 17%   Ratio: 2:1

Applesauce Yogurt Muffins

MAKES 12 MUFFINS / PREP TIME: 10 MINUTES / COOK TIME: 18 MINUTES

Under 30 Minutes • Make Ahead *Muffins are a popular grab-and-go breakfast for anyone who is chronically overscheduled or culinarily challenged. Fortunately these sweet beauties are low calorie and have the perfect combination of fat and protein to get you through the morning. You can replace the Greek yogurt with sour cream if you want to add a little more fat to your meal.*

1. Preheat the oven to 350°F.

2. Line a 12-cup muffin pan with paper liners, and set aside.

3. In a large bowl, stir together the almond flour, flaxseed meal, baking powder, stevia, cinnamon, nutmeg, ginger, and salt.

4. In a medium bowl, whisk together the eggs, yogurt, applesauce, butter, and vanilla.

5. Add the wet ingredients to the dry ingredients, and stir to blend.

6. Spoon the muffin batter into the muffin cups evenly.

7. Bake until the muffins are golden and a knife inserted in the center of one comes out clean, about 18 minutes.

8. Cool the muffins on wire racks, and serve.

PER SERVING: CALORIES: 94 / FAT: 8G / TOTAL CARBS: 3G
FIBER: 1G / NET CARBS: 2G / SUGAR: 2G / PROTEIN: 3G

Fat 75% / Carbs 12% / Protein 13%   Ratio: 3:1

½ cup almond flour

2 tablespoons flaxseed meal

½ teaspoon baking powder

½ teaspoon stevia

½ teaspoon ground cinnamon

½ teaspoon ground nutmeg

¼ teaspoon ground ginger

¼ teaspoon sea salt

3 large eggs

½ cup plain Greek yogurt

½ cup unsweetened applesauce

3 tablespoons butter, melted

1 teaspoon pure vanilla extract

IN MENU FOR WEEK:

2

A CLOSER LOOK: *Flaxseed is popular with any group looking to add protein and healthy omega-3 fatty acids to their diet, such as bodybuilders or professional athletes. Heating it in the oven will not reduce the omega-3 fatty acid (alpha-linolenic acid) in this powerhouse seed, so flaxseed is a wonderful addition to baked goods.*

"Cornbread" Muffins

MAKES 12 MUFFINS / PREP TIME: 10 MINUTES / COOK TIME: 20 MINUTES

2 cups almond flour

2 tablespoons flaxseed meal

2 teaspoons baking powder

6 large eggs, beaten

½ cup plain Greek yogurt

½ teaspoon stevia

IN MENU FOR WEEK:

4

Under 30 Minutes • Make Ahead *This is not real cornbread, but the flaxseed meal and almond flour create a very comparable texture to these muffins. Similar to traditional cornbread, you can jazz up this recipe with Cheddar, minced jalapeño peppers, and chopped cooked bacon. The batter can also be baked in a loaf pan if you increase the cooking time to 45 minutes.*

1. Preheat the oven to 350°F.

2. Line a 12-cup muffin pan with paper liners, and set aside.

3. In a large bowl, stir together the almond flour, flaxseed meal, and baking powder.

4. Stir in the eggs, yogurt, and stevia until the batter is smooth.

5. Spoon the batter evenly among the muffin cups.

6. Bake until the muffins are lightly browned and firm, about 15 minutes.

7. Cool the muffins on wire racks, and serve.

PER SERVING: CALORIES: 163 / FAT: 13G / TOTAL CARBS: 5G
FIBER: 2G / NET CARBS: 3G / SUGAR: 1G / PROTEIN: 4G

Fat 70% / Carbs 16% / Protein 14%   Ratio: 3:1

Buttery Coconut Bread

MAKES 16 SLICES / PREP TIME: 10 MINUTES / COOK TIME: 35 MINUTES

Make Ahead *The ingredients and presentation of this cake might seem plain, but the flavor is as buttery and rich as a classic pound cake. One small slice will fill you up and keep your energy levels high all morning. Try chilling the coconut bread in the refrigerator to firm it up and toasting a slice for a truly divine treat.*

1. Preheat the oven to 350°F.
2. Lightly grease an 8-by-4-inch loaf pan with butter, and set aside.
3. In a medium bowl, whisk together the melted butter, eggs, and stevia until well blended.
4. In a small bowl, stir together the almond flour, coconut flour, and baking powder until mixed.
5. Add the coconut flour mixture to the egg mixture, and stir to combine.
6. Stir in the vanilla.
7. Spoon the batter into the loaf pan, and bake the bread until it is golden brown and pulls away from the sides of the pan, about 35 minutes.
8. Cool the bread in the loaf pan for 15 minutes, and then turn the bread out onto a wire rack to cool completely.
9. Store in a sealed container in the fridge for up to 1 week.

PER SERVING (1 SLICE): CALORIES: 107 / FAT: 9G / TOTAL CARBS: 4G
FIBER: 2G / NET CARBS: 2G / SUGAR: 1G / PROTEIN: 4G

Fat 74% / Carbs 12% / Protein 14%   Ratio: 2:1

½ cup butter, melted, plus more for greasing

6 large eggs

½ teaspoon stevia

1 cup almond flour

½ cup coconut flour

1 teaspoon baking powder

1 teaspoon pure vanilla extract

IN MENU FOR WEEKS:

A CLOSER LOOK: *Coconut flour is the solid left over when coconut milk is made from grinding up the coconut and adding water. Coconut flour can be substituted for regular flour in a 1:4 ratio as long as you increase the liquid in the recipe as well, because coconut flour sucks up moisture like a sponge. In general, you need to add 1 cup of liquid (such as coconut milk or heavy cream) or 6 eggs per cup of coconut flour.*

Spanakopita Omelet

SERVES 4 / PREP TIME: 15 MINUTES / COOK TIME: 30 MINUTES

5 tablespoons butter, divided

2 teaspoons minced garlic

3 cups white mushrooms

10 cups spinach

12 eggs, divided

1 cup feta cheese

Sea salt

Freshly ground black pepper

IN MENU FOR WEEKS:

Spinach, feta, and mushrooms are the base ingredients found in Greece's famous dish spanakopita, or spinach pie. Traditional feta cheese is created from 30 percent goat's milk mixed with sheep's milk, and the flavor and texture of the cheese depends on the area where the animals graze. This recipe is best with a drier, more robust cheese packed in brine.

1. In a large skillet over medium heat, melt 2 tablespoons of butter.

2. Sauté the garlic until it is softened, about 3 minutes.

3. Add the mushrooms and sauté until they are light golden, about 5 minutes.

4. Melt 2 more tablespoons of butter in the skillet, and stir in the spinach.

5. Sauté until the greens are wilted, about 3 minutes.

6. Remove the skillet from the heat, and transfer the spinach, mushrooms, and garlic to a large bowl, leaving any excess liquid in the skillet.

7. Wipe out the skillet, and place it back on the heat.

8. Melt 1 tablespoon of butter in the skillet.

9. Crack 3 eggs into a small bowl, and whisk to blend.

10. Pour the eggs into the skillet, and swirl the pan so that the eggs keep moving for about 30 seconds to set on the bottom.

11. Lift the edges of the cooked egg to allow the raw egg to flow underneath until the omelet is cooked through, about 3 minutes.

12. Spoon ¼ of the spinach mixture onto the cooked egg, and sprinkle with ¼ cup of the feta.

13. Flip one side over, slide the omelet onto a serving plate, and season with salt and pepper.

14. Repeat to create 3 more omelets, and serve.

_____

PER SERVING: CALORIES: 548 / FAT: 45G / TOTAL CARBS: 8G
FIBER: 2G / NET CARBS: 6G / SUGAR: 4G / PROTEIN: 26G

Fat 75% / Carbs 6% / Protein 19%   Ratio: 2:1

Fluffy Baked Omelet with Pancetta and Swiss Cheese

SERVES 4 / PREP TIME: 10 MINUTES / COOK TIME: 40 MINUTES

1 tablespoon butter, plus more for greasing

1 cup diced pancetta

10 large eggs

1 cup coconut milk

1 cup shredded Swiss cheese

2 teaspoons chopped chives

Pinch sea salt

Freshly ground black pepper

IN MENU FOR WEEKS:

TRY INSTEAD: *Pancetta has a wonderful salty taste that adds depth to the flavor of this omelet, but bacon, ham, or peameal bacon would work nicely as well. Substitute in the same quantities as the pancetta if you want to try other cured meats.*

The best Swiss cheese for this simple omelet is Emmental, which has the distinctive holes that most people think of when Swiss cheese is mentioned. The holes are actually quite difficult to produce and require a complicated fermentation process. This cheese has a smooth flavor, almost fruity, and a firm, fine-grained texture.

1. Preheat the oven to 350°F.
2. Lightly grease a 9-by-9-inch baking dish with butter, and set aside.
3. In a large skillet over medium-high heat, melt the butter.
4. Cook the pancetta, stirring, until it is crispy, about 4 minutes.
5. Remove the skillet from the heat, and transfer the pancetta to a medium bowl.
6. Add the eggs, coconut milk, cheese, and chives to the bowl, and whisk to blend.
7. Season the egg mixture with salt and pepper.
8. Pour the egg mixture into the baking dish, and place it in the center of the oven.
9. Bake the omelet until it is set, puffy, and golden, about 30 minutes, and serve.

PER SERVING: CALORIES: 496 / FAT: 41G / TOTAL CARBS: 6G
FIBER: 1G / NET CARBS: 5G / SUGAR: 3G / PROTEIN: 27G

Fat 74% / Carbs 5% / Protein 21%   Ratio: 2:1

Jalapeño Frittata

SERVES 4 / PREP TIME: 15 MINUTES / COOK TIME: 30 MINUTES

Make Ahead *Hot peppers come in many different shapes, colors, and degrees of heat. There is a measurement called the Scoville scale that rates peppers in Scoville heat units (SHU) to indicate capsaicin concentration, or hotness. Jalapeño peppers rate as quite mild on this scale, only 1,000 to 4,000 SHU. If you want a true palate-scorching breakfast, substitute serrano peppers or habaneros in smaller quantities.*

1. Preheat the oven to 350°F.

2. Lightly grease an 8-by-8-inch baking dish with butter, and set aside.

3. In a small bowl, stir together the cream cheese, 1 chopped jalapeño pepper, and ¼ cup of Cheddar until blended. Set aside.

4. In a medium bowl, whisk together the eggs, milk, cream, salt, and chili powder.

5. Using a tablespoon, drop clumps of the cream cheese mixture into the baking dish until all of the mixture is used up; do not spread the mixture out.

6. Pour the egg mixture into the baking dish.

7. Top the egg evenly with the remaining jalapeño pepper and ½ cup of Cheddar.

8. Bake until the eggs are set and the cheese is golden and bubbly, about 30 minutes.

9. Cut the frittata into 4 generous pieces, and serve.

PER SERVING: CALORIES: 362 / FAT: 31G / TOTAL CARBS: 3G
FIBER: 0G / NET CARBS: 3G / SUGAR: 1G / PROTEIN: 17G

Fat 77% / Carbs 4% / Protein 19% Ratio: 2:1

Butter, for greasing

6 ounces cream cheese, softened

2 jalapeño peppers, chopped, divided

¾ cup shredded aged Cheddar cheese, divided

6 large eggs

½ cup unsweetened almond milk

2 tablespoons heavy (whipping) cream

Pinch sea salt

Pinch chili powder

IN MENU FOR WEEKS:

Skillet-Baked Eggs with Yogurt and Spinach

SERVES 4 / PREP TIME: 10 MINUTES / COOK TIME: 25 MINUTES

½ cup plain Greek-style yogurt

1 teaspoon freshly squeezed lemon juice

¼ teaspoon chili powder

2 tablespoons butter

2 tablespoons extra-virgin olive oil

½ white onion, diced

8 cups spinach

4 large eggs

1 teaspoon chopped fresh cilantro, for topping

Eggs are a staple of the ketogenic diet, but enjoying them in a variety of preparations is key to making sure you don't get bored. In this dish, the yolks will crack open at the first touch of your fork, creating a rich sauce that blends deliciously with the yogurt and spinach.

1. In a small bowl, stir together the yogurt, lemon juice, and chili powder, and set aside.

2. Preheat the oven to 350°F.

3. In a large, ovenproof skillet over medium heat, heat the butter and olive oil. Add the onion, and sauté until soft, about 5 minutes.

4. Stir in the spinach, and sauté, tossing frequently, until wilted, about 5 minutes.

5. Push the spinach to the side of the skillet, and spoon out any extra liquid.

6. Arrange the spinach so it covers the entire bottom of the skillet, and use a spoon to make 4 wells in the greens.

7. Break the eggs into the wells, and place the skillet in the oven.

8. Bake until the whites are set, about 10 minutes.

9. Spoon the yogurt mixture over the eggs, top with the cilantro, and serve.

PER SERVING: CALORIES: 241 / FAT: 23G / TOTAL CARBS: 5G
FIBER: 2G / NET CARBS: 3G / SUGAR: 2G / PROTEIN: 9G

Fat 80% / Carbs 5% / Protein 15%   Ratio: 2:1

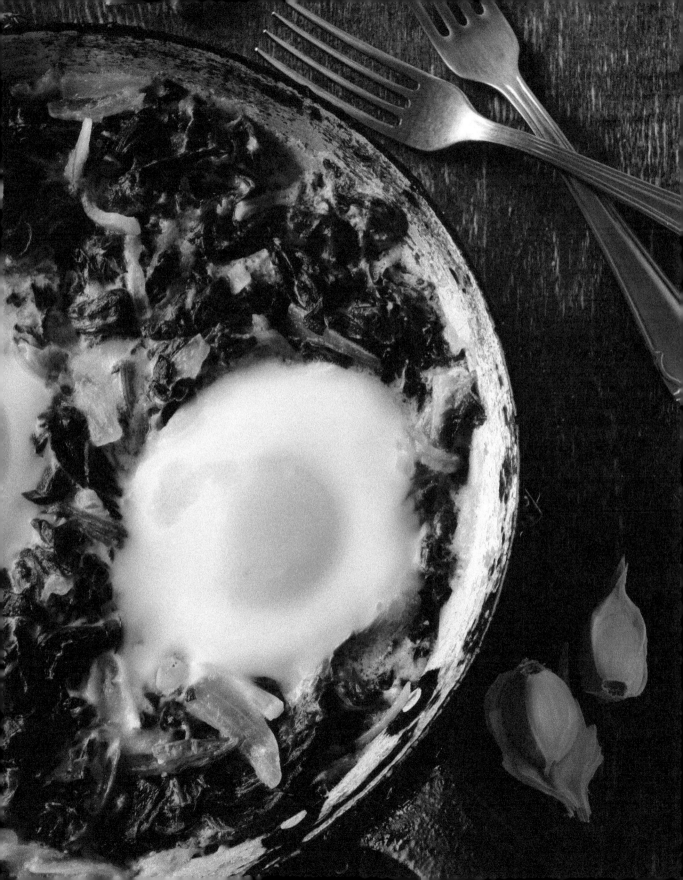

Egg Breakfast Muffins

SERVES 4 / PREP TIME: 5 MINUTES / COOK TIME: 16 MINUTES

1 tablespoon butter, for greasing

6 large eggs

1 cup heavy (whipping) cream

½ cup plus 2 tablespoons Cheddar cheese, divided

5 slices cooked bacon, chopped

½ teaspoon chopped cilantro

Pinch salt

Pinch freshly ground black pepper

IN MENU FOR WEEK:

2

KITCHEN HACK: *You will be using bacon regularly in a ketogenic lifestyle because it provides a good ratio of fat and protein. Cooked bacon will keep for at least 1 week in the refrigerator, so cook up an entire pack so you can save time when you need to add this product to your recipes in cooked form.*

Under 30 Minutes • Make Ahead *These pretty, cheesy muffins are actually quiches baked in a muffin pan without the crust. You can eat them hot out of the oven or chilled, depending on your schedule. These muffins also freeze beautifully, so whip up a double batch for easy meals all month.*

1. Preheat the oven to 350°F.

2. Lightly grease 8 cups of a muffin pan with the butter, and set aside.

3. In a medium bowl, whisk together the eggs, cream, ½ cup of Cheddar, bacon, and cilantro.

4. Season the egg mixture with salt and pepper.

5. Evenly pour the egg mixture into the muffin cups.

6. Bake the muffins until they are cooked through and lightly browned, about 15 minutes.

7. Remove the muffin pan from the oven, and change the oven heat to broil.

8. Sprinkle the remaining 2 tablespoons of Cheddar onto the muffins, broil until the cheese is melted and bubbly, about 1 minute, and serve.

PER SERVING (2 MUFFINS): CALORIES: 346 / FAT: 31G
TOTAL CARBS: 2G / FIBER: 0G / NET CARBS: 2G
SUGAR: 1G / PROTEIN: 15G

Fat 79% / Carbs 2% / Protein 19%   Ratio: 2:1

Simple Scrambled Eggs

SERVES 4 / PREP TIME: 5 MINUTES / COOK TIME: 5 MINUTES

Under 30 Minutes *Scrambled eggs are often overcooked and grainy when you get them in restaurants or huge heaps in chafing dishes during events. Well-cooked scrambled eggs should be moist, large curds with a lovely, creamy texture and a hint of seasoning. The trick is to avoid high heat or overworking the eggs as they firm up in the skillet.*

1. In a large bowl, whisk together the eggs and heavy cream. Set aside.

2. Place a large skillet over medium heat and melt the butter.

3. Pour the egg mixture into the skillet and use a plastic spatula to pull the eggs into the center of the skillet as it cooks.

4. Continue to scrape the skillet, creating moist, fluffy egg curds, until the eggs are just cooked, about 4 minutes.

5. Stir in the tarragon, season the eggs with salt and pepper, and serve.

10 large eggs

½ cup heavy (whipping) cream

2 tablespoons butter

1 teaspoon chopped tarragon

Sea salt

Freshly ground black pepper

IN MENU FOR WEEK:

1

PER SERVING: CALORIES: 282 / FAT: 24G / TOTAL CARBS: 2G
FIBER: 0G / NET CARBS: 2G / SUGAR: 1G / PROTEIN: 15G

Fat 76% / Carbs 3% / Protein 21%   Ratio: 2:1

Breakfast "Sandwich"

SERVES 4 / PREP TIME: 15 MINUTES / COOK TIME: 15 MINUTES

Peameal bacon, a cross between traditional smoked bacon and ham, is a lightly brined pork loin that is rolled in cornmeal. This delectable meat does not crisp up in the skillet, so be prepared for a juicy, slightly sweet base for your sandwich.

1. In a large skillet over medium-high heat, heat the olive oil. Sauté the jalapeño peppers, bell peppers, and leeks until tender, about 4 minutes.

2. Transfer the pepper-leek mixture to a small bowl, and set aside.

3. Wipe out the skillet, and place it back over medium-high heat. Add 1½ tablespoons of butter.

4. Cook the peameal bacon, turning once, until it is browned and cooked through, about 5 minutes total.

5. Remove the bacon from the skillet, and place 1 piece on each plate.

6. Place 1 tablespoon of cream cheese in the middle of each piece of bacon.

7. Wipe the skillet out, and place it back over medium-high heat.

8. Add the remaining 1½ tablespoons of butter, and fry the eggs until the whites are firm and the edges are lacy and brown, about 4 minutes.

9. Top the cream cheese and bacon with 1 egg per plate, and season with salt and pepper.

10. Divide the pepper-leek mixture evenly among the eggs, top each dish with a sprinkle of thyme, and serve.

1 tablespoon extra-virgin olive oil

2 jalapeño peppers, seeded and chopped

1 red bell pepper, chopped

½ leek, julienned

3 tablespoons butter, divided

4 (3.5 ounce) peameal bacon slices

4 tablespoons cream cheese

4 large eggs

Sea salt

Freshly ground black pepper

1 teaspoon chopped fresh thyme, for garnish

IN MENU FOR WEEK:

 2

PER SERVING: CALORIES: 338 / FAT: 26G / TOTAL CARBS: 7G
FIBER: 2G / NET CARBS: 5G / SUGAR: 2G / PROTEIN: 22G

Fat 70% / Carbs 5% / Protein 25%   Ratio: 3:1

Corned Beef Breakfast Hash

SERVES 4 / PREP TIME: 20 MINUTES / COOK TIME: 20 MINUTES

3 tablespoons butter, divided

8 ounces corned beef, chopped

2 cups chopped cauliflower

2 scallions, chopped

Sea salt

Freshly ground black pepper

4 large eggs

2 tablespoons parsley, for garnish

IN MENU FOR WEEK:

1

TRY INSTEAD: *The cauliflower adds satisfying bulk to this dish and an acceptable amount of carbs. You can also use shredded green cabbage for a more traditional corned beef hash variation. Do not use red cabbage in this recipe unless you enjoy a purple-hued breakfast.*

Corned beef is preserved meat that does not contain any sort of corn at all. The term "corned" refers to the kernels of rock salt that are heaped over the meat in large crocks during the curing process. This type of meat was often a staple food for sailors or travelers because it did not spoil during long trips.

1. In a large skillet over medium-high heat, melt 1½ tablespoons of butter.

2. Sauté the corned beef for 5 minutes, until it is heated through and the fat renders out of the meat.

3. Stir in the cauliflower, and sauté until the cauliflower is tender and lightly caramelized, about 10 minutes.

4. Add the scallions, and sauté 1 minute.

5. Season the hash with salt and pepper.

6. Remove the skillet from the heat, and set aside.

7. In another large skillet over medium-high heat, melt the remaining 1½ tablespoons of butter.

8. Fry the eggs sunny-side up in the butter until the whites are cooked through, about 4 minutes.

9. Serve the hash topped with 1 egg per person and garnished with fresh parsley.

PER SERVING: CALORIES: 251 / FAT: 21G / TOTAL CARBS: 4G
FIBER: 2G / NET CARBS: 2G / SUGAR: 2G / PROTEIN: 13G

Fat 72% / Carbs 6% / Protein 22%   Ratio: 2:1

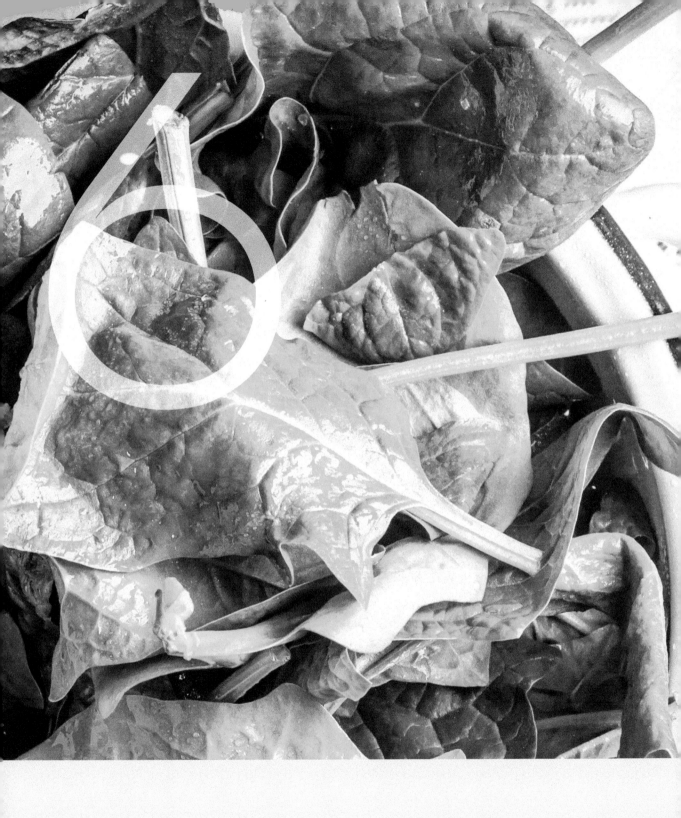

SMOOTHIES

Creamy Kale Smoothie

SERVES 2 / PREP TIME: 10 MINUTES

¾ cup unsweetened almond milk

¼ cup unsweetened apple juice

½ cup lightly steamed kale

¼ cup cream cheese

1 tablespoon hemp seeds

2 (7g) stevia packets

2 cups ice cubes

Under 30 Minutes • One Pot *Kale is often used in smoothies for its nutrition profile and its ability to combine well with many different ingredients. Kale can help fight cancer, support cardiovascular health, and reduce inflammation in the body. You can use kale raw, but cooking this fabulous green lightly boosts its health benefits. For example, steamed kale lowers cholesterol levels more than raw.*

1. In a blender, blend the almond milk, apple juice, kale, cream cheese, hemp seeds, and stevia until combined.
2. Add the ice, and blend until smooth and thick.
3. Pour the smoothie into 2 glasses, and serve.

PER SERVING: CALORIES: 152 / FAT: 13G / TOTAL CARBS: 4G
FIBER: 1G / NET CARBS: 3G / SUGAR: 0G / PROTEIN: 5G

Fat 78% / Carbs 7% / Protein 15%   Ratio: 2:1

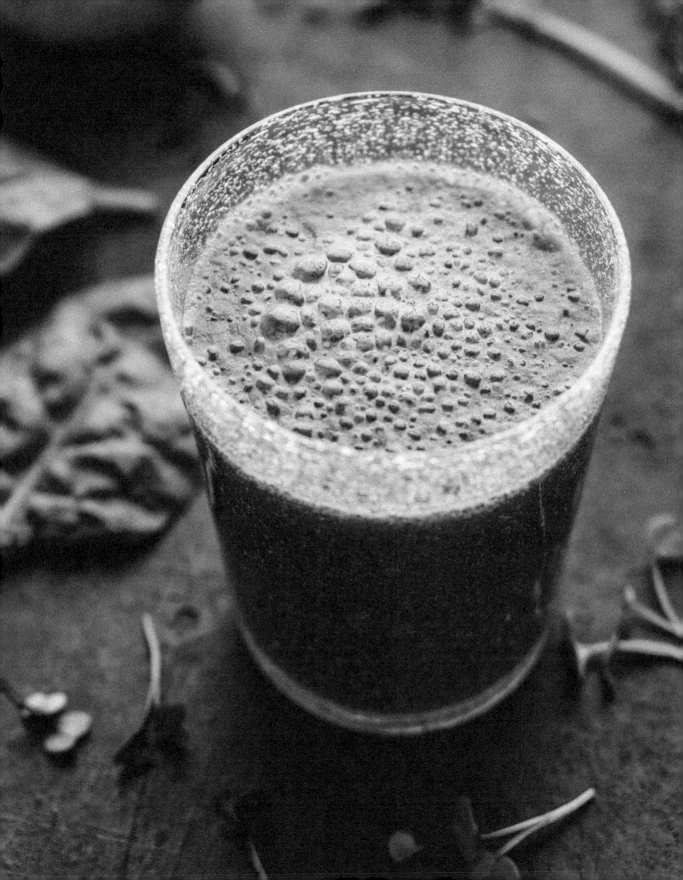

Cheesecake Smoothie

SERVES 2 / PREP TIME: 10 MINUTES

¾ cup unsweetened almond milk

¼ cup Greek yogurt

2 tablespoons cream cheese

1 tablespoon heavy (whipping) cream

2 (7g) stevia packets

2 cups ice cubes

TRY INSTEAD: *If you have some carb grams left in your daily totals, this smoothie is spectacular with a handful of frozen strawberries, raspberries, or peaches. Try ¼ cup of cocoa powder to make a chocolate-cheesecake flavor for a real treat.*

Under 30 Minutes • One Pot *Cheesecake conjures up visions of sublime indulgence, almost sinful in character. The richness, the excess, the silky-smooth texture of this dessert is duplicated in this icy smoothie. For extra richness and fat grams, add a couple extra tablespoons of cream cheese to your blender.*

1. In a blender, blend the almond milk, yogurt, cream cheese, cream, and stevia until combined.

2. Add the ice, and blend until smooth and thick.

3. Pour the smoothie into 2 glasses, and serve.

PER SERVING: CALORIES: 113 / FAT: 9G / TOTAL CARBS: 2G
FIBER: 0G / NET CARBS: 2G / SUGAR: 1G / PROTEIN: 5G

Fat 79% / Carbs 3% / Protein 18%   Ratio: 2:1

Chocolate-Mint Smoothie

SERVES 2 / PREP TIME: 10 MINUTES

Under 30 Minutes • One Pot *This classic taste combination brings the richness of chocolate together with the sharpness of fresh mint. The best mint to use for this recipe is peppermint rather than spearmint because it has a stronger flavor, and always purchase or harvest young, small leaves to avoid bitterness. Mint is a folk remedy for stomach complaints, headache, and sleep problems.*

1 cup unsweetened almond milk

2 tablespoons almond butter

2 tablespoons cocoa powder

1 teaspoon chopped fresh mint

2 (7g) stevia packets

1 cup ice cubes

1. In a blender, blend the almond milk, almond butter, cocoa powder, mint, and stevia until combined.

2. Add the ice, and blend until smooth.

3. Pour the smoothie into 2 glasses, and serve.

PER SERVING: CALORIES: 129 / FAT: 11G / TOTAL CARBS: 6G
FIBER: 3G / NET CARBS: 3G / SUGAR: 0G / PROTEIN: 5G

Fat 76% / Carbs 15% / Protein 9%   Ratio: 2:1

A CLOSER LOOK: *Almond butter can be a little more expensive than the perpetual favorite, peanut butter; however, almond butter is packed with vitamin E and low in saturated fat. Almond butter is a good source of protein, calcium, iron, and magnesium.*

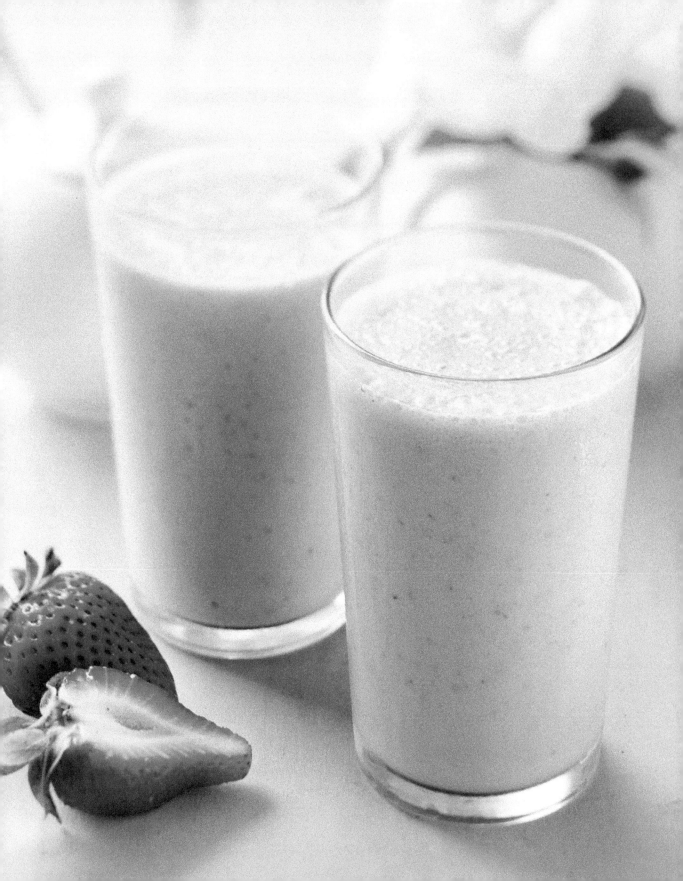

Tropical Smoothie

SERVES 2 / PREP TIME: 10 MINUTES

Under 30 Minutes • One Pot *Banana extract often gets poor reviews because the flavor of some products is cloying and has a strange chemical component. Finding an acceptable extract can be a matter of personal taste as well as trial and error. If you can find banana extract powder, created from dehydrated or freeze-dried banana peel and fruit, you might be more pleased with the taste.*

½ cup coconut milk

¼ cup plain Greek yogurt

2 tablespoons hemp seeds

2 (7g) stevia packets

1 teaspoon banana extract

2 strawberries

2 cups ice cubes

1. In a blender, blend the coconut milk, yogurt, hemp seeds, stevia, banana extract, and strawberries until combined.

2. Add the ice, and blend until smooth.

3. Pour the smoothie into 2 glasses, and serve.

PER SERVING: CALORIES: 201 / FAT: 18G / TOTAL CARBS: 5G
FIBER: 2G / NET CARBS: 3G / SUGAR: 3G / PROTEIN: 7G

Fat 78% / Carbs 8% / Protein 14%   Ratio: 2:1

Avocado-Lime Smoothie

SERVES 2 / PREP TIME: 10 MINUTES

1 cup unsweetened almond milk

Juice and zest of 1 lime

¼ avocado

2 tablespoons hemp seeds

1 teaspoon pure vanilla extract

2 (7g) stevia packets

2 cups ice cubes

Under 30 Minutes • One Pot *Avocado can be a difficult fruit to store after you cut it open for your recipes, like in this case, when you are left with three-quarters of the flesh after making the smoothie. Avocado often oxidizes into a brown, slimy mess even when it is wrapped in plastic and stored in the refrigerator. The best way to keep leftover avocado fresh and green is to place it in a sealed container with half a cut onion. The sulfur from the onion prevents oxidization.*

1. In a blender, blend the almond milk, lime juice, lime zest, avocado, hemp seeds, vanilla, and stevia until combined.

2. Add the ice cubes, and blend until smooth and thick.

3. Pour the smoothie into 2 glasses, and serve.

PER SERVING: CALORIES: 114 / FAT: 10G / TOTAL CARBS: 5G
FIBER: 3G / NET CARBS: 2G / SUGAR: 0G / PROTEIN: 4G

Fat 75% / Carbs 16% / Protein 9%   Ratio: 2:1

Cucumber Green Smoothie

SERVES 2 / PREP TIME: 10 MINUTES

Under 30 Minutes • One Pot *Green smoothies are touted as the best breakfast and snack choice because they are so nutritious. Most dark leafy greens, like the spinach in this drink, are packed with vitamins A, D, E, and K, which are all fat soluble. This means these vitamins are readily available to the body when combined with the coconut oil and tahini in this recipe.*

1. In a blender, blend the cucumber, spinach, coconut milk, egg white protein powder, tahini, and coconut oil until combined.

2. Add the ice cubes, and blend until smooth and thick.

3. Pour the smoothie into 2 glasses, and serve.

1 English cucumber

1 cup spinach

½ cup coconut milk

3 tablespoons egg white protein powder

1 tablespoon tahini

1 teaspoon coconut oil

2 cups ice cubes

IN MENU FOR WEEKS:

 2   4

PER SERVING: CALORIES: 258 / FAT: 21G / TOTAL CARBS: 11G
FIBER: 3G / NET CARBS: 8G / SUGAR: 5G / PROTEIN: 10G

Fat 72% / Carbs 15% / Protein 13%   Ratio: 2:1

Peanut Butter Smoothie

SERVES 2 / PREP TIME: 10 MINUTES

1 cup unsweetened
almond milk

½ cup coconut milk

3 tablespoons natural
peanut butter

1 teaspoon pure vanilla
extract

2 (7g) stevia packets

2 cups ice cubes

Under 30 Minutes • One Pot *Most people have a handy jar of peanut butter in their pantry, but it is probably "regular" peanut butter rather than a natural product. Regular peanut butter has added vegetable oil to prevent the separation of solids and oils as well as a significant amount of sugar. This recipe is best if you use a peanuts-only butter that has been stirred just before using to ensure an even texture and oil distribution.*

1. In a blender, blend the almond milk, coconut milk, peanut butter, vanilla, and stevia until combined.

2. Add the ice, and blend until smooth and thick.

3. Pour the smoothie into 2 glasses, and serve.

PER SERVING: CALORIES: 309 / FAT: 27G / TOTAL CARBS: 8G
FIBER: 4G / NET CARBS: 4G / SUGAR: 4G / PROTEIN: 9G

Fat 78% / Carbs 10% / Protein 12%   Ratio: 3:1

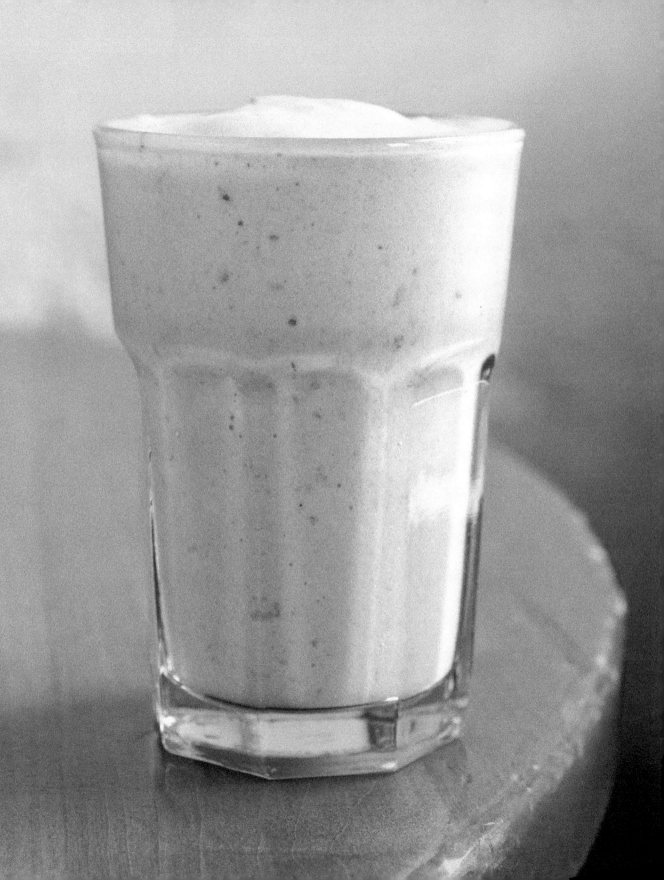

Lemon Smoothie

SERVES 2 / PREP TIME: 10 MINUTES

1 cup unsweetened
almond milk

½ cup coconut milk

2 tablespoons egg white
protein powder

1 teaspoon pure vanilla
extract

1 teaspoon lemon extract

2 (7g) stevia packets

2 cups ice cubes

IN MENU FOR WEEK:

1

A CLOSER LOOK: *Egg white
protein powder is one
of the best ways to add
protein to your diet without
any unwanted additives.
This powder contains high-
quality protein, is lactose
free, and has very low levels
of carbohydrates. Egg white
protein powder is also a
good source of vitamins A,
B, D, and E.*

Under 30 Minutes • One Pot *Lemon extract is often used instead of
lemon juice because it adds strong lemon flavor to recipes without
any sourness. Lemon extract is made from the rind of lemons,
not the flesh, and is a great substitute for lemon zest rather than
lemon juice. So if you do not have lemon extract, add a teaspoon
of freshly grated lemon zest to this smoothie to duplicate the taste.*

1. In a blender, blend the almond milk, coconut milk,
   egg white powder, vanilla, lemon extract, and stevia
   until combined.

2. Add the ice, and blend until smooth and thick.

3. Pour the smoothie into 2 glasses, and serve.

PER SERVING: CALORIES: 172 / FAT: 14G / TOTAL CARBS: 4G
FIBER: 1G / NET CARBS: 3G / SUGAR: 2G / PROTEIN: 6G

Fat 72% / Carbs 12% / Protein 16%   Ratio: 2:1

Vanilla Bean Smoothie

SERVES 2 / PREP TIME: 10 MINUTES

Under 30 Minutes • One Pot *Coconut oil has reached super-food status in the last few decades after spending years on the do-not-eat list for many healthy diet enthusiasts. The high saturated fat content of this oil was linked erroneously with heart disease until it was reported that two-thirds of the saturated fat in coconut oil is a medium chain fatty acid (MCFA). MCFAs are easily digested and are converted by the liver to energy rather than stored as fat.*

1. In a blender, blend the almond milk, avocado, egg white powder, coconut oil, vanilla bean seeds, and cinnamon until combined.

2. Add the ice, and blend until smooth and thick.

3. Pour the smoothie into 2 glasses, and serve.

PER SERVING: CALORIES: 158 / FAT: 13G / TOTAL CARBS: 5G
FIBER: 4G / NET CARBS: 1G / SUGAR: 1G / PROTEIN: 6G

Fat 74% / Carbs 12% / Protein 14%   Ratio: 2:1

1 cup almond milk

½ avocado

2 tablespoons egg white protein powder

1 teaspoon coconut oil

Seeds of 1 vanilla bean

¼ teaspoon ground cinnamon

2 cups ice cubes

TRY INSTEAD: *Vanilla beans add a rich, pure flavor to recipes, but if you do not have these shiny dark beans on hand, you can use 2 teaspoons of vanilla extract instead. Make sure you purchase pure vanilla extract instead of artificial to get the best results and no bitter aftertaste.*

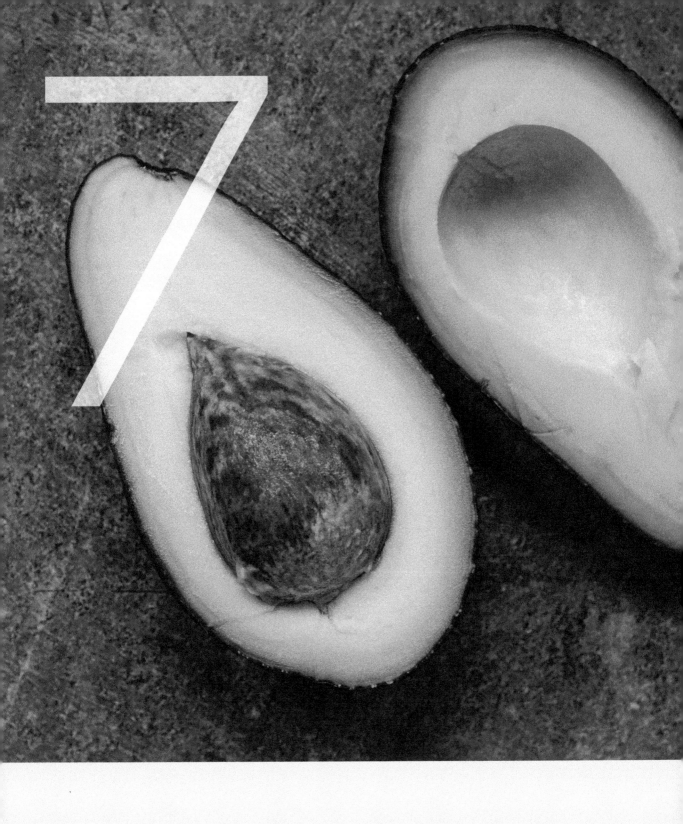

SALADS, SOUPS, AND STEWS

Cobb Salad

SERVES 4 / PREP TIME: 15 MINUTES

FOR THE DRESSING

2 tablespoons extra-virgin olive oil

1 tablespoon balsamic vinegar

1 teaspoon freshly squeezed lemon juice

1 teaspoon Dijon mustard

½ teaspoon garlic powder

Sea salt

Freshly ground black pepper

FOR THE SALAD

2 cups shredded romaine lettuce

6 cherry tomatoes, halved

2 hard-boiled eggs, chopped

½ cup blue cheese, crumbled

½ avocado, diced

6 bacon slices, chopped

IN MENU FOR WEEKS:

KITCHEN HACK: *Hard-boil an entire carton to keep in the fridge for recipes that need cooked eggs, for egg salad, and as a handy, quick snack. You can store them for up to one week in the refrigerator.*

Under 30 Minutes *The origin of many signature dishes is often fuzzy, so it is wonderful to know definitively that the Cobb salad was created by the owner of the Brown Derby restaurant in Hollywood in the 1930s. Bob Cobb threw together the ingredients of the salad as a late-night snack while in the company of his peer Sid Grauman, who owned the famous Grauman's Chinese Theatre. The salad was so delicious that Mr. Grauman asked for a Cobb salad the next day, and the dish joined the menu permanently. Try adding grilled chicken and a handful of pumpkin or sunflower seeds for a more substantial salad.*

TO MAKE THE DRESSING

1. In a small bowl, whisk together the olive oil, balsamic vinegar, lemon juice, Dijon mustard, and garlic powder.

2. Season the dressing with salt and pepper, and set aside.

TO MAKE THE SALAD

1. In a medium bowl, toss the lettuce well with the dressing.

2. Arrange the dressed salad on 4 plates.

3. Top each salad with cherry tomatoes, chopped eggs, blue cheese, avocado, and bacon bits, and serve.

PER SERVING: CALORIES: 209 / FAT: 16G / TOTAL CARBS: 7G
FIBER: 3G / NET CARBS: 4G / SUGAR: 4G / PROTEIN: 11G

Fat 70% / Carbs 9% / Protein 21%   Ratio: 2:1

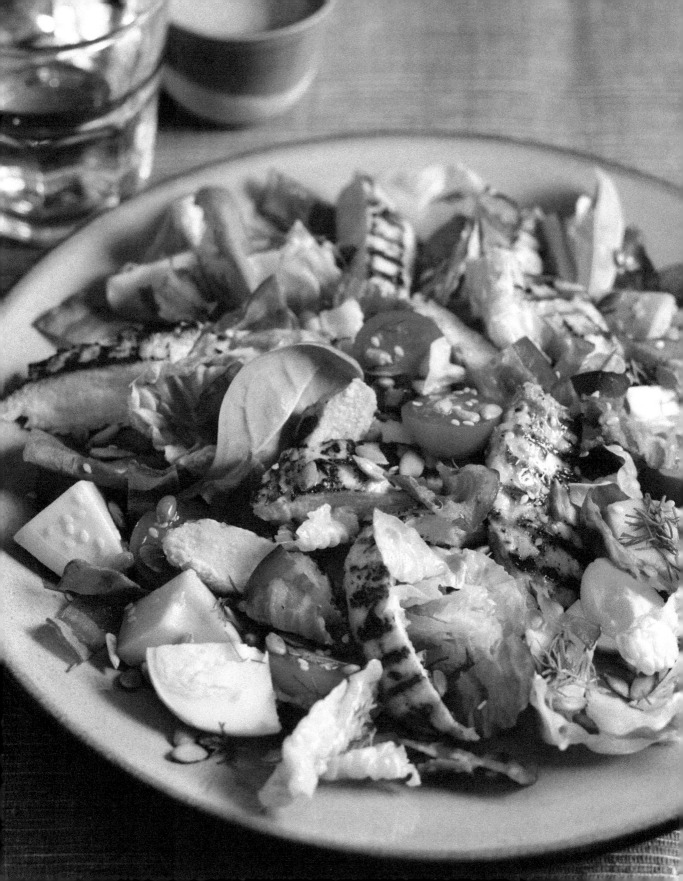

Walnut-Fennel Salad with Sherry Vinaigrette

SERVES 4 / PREP TIME: 25 MINUTES

FOR THE VINAIGRETTE

⅓ cup walnut oil

2 tablespoons sherry vinegar

1 tablespoon minced shallot

1 teaspoon chopped fresh thyme

FOR THE SALAD

2 cups shredded arugula

1 cup shredded romaine

½ cup thinly sliced fennel

½ avocado, diced

½ cup walnuts, chopped

3 ounces goat cheese, crumbled

IN MENU FOR WEEKS:

Under 30 Minutes *Fennel is related to parsley and carrot but looks like a bulbous bunch of celery topped with feathery fronds. The best fennel is found from fall to very early spring when there are no flowering buds, which indicate the vegetable is past its prime and woody. Eat your fennel within a couple days of purchase because it loses its flavor the longer it spends in the refrigerator.*

TO MAKE THE VINAIGRETTE

1. In a small bowl, whisk together the walnut oil, vinegar, shallot, and thyme.

2. Set aside.

TO MAKE THE SALAD

1. In a medium bowl, toss together the arugula, romaine, and fennel with the dressing until the ingredients are coated.

2. Arrange the greens and fennel on 4 plates, top each salad evenly with avocado, walnuts, and goat cheese, and serve.

PER SERVING: CALORIES: 384 / FAT: 34G / TOTAL CARBS: 8G
FIBER: 5G / NET CARBS: 3G / SUGAR: 1G / PROTEIN: 16G

Fat 78% / Carbs 6% / Protein 16%   Ratio: 2:1

Asian Shrimp Salad

SERVES 4 / PREP TIME: 25 MINUTES

Under 30 Minutes *The spicy sauce, crisp vegetables, and sweet shrimp combine beautifully in this meal-size salad. You can certainly enjoy this dish as an appetizer, but the strong flavors stand alone and could overwhelm the palate if eaten first. If you want to make the salad ahead of time, substitute shredded cabbage for the romaine because it holds its texture better as it sits in the dressing.*

TO MAKE THE DRESSING

1. In a small bowl, whisk together the olive oil, lime juice, soy sauce, sambal oelek, fish sauce, and stevia.
2. Set aside.

TO MAKE THE SALAD

1. In a large bowl, toss together the romaine, snow peas, red pepper, and cilantro.
2. Add the dressing, and toss to coat.
3. Arrange the salad on 4 plates, and evenly divide the shrimp among the salads.
4. Top each salad with peanuts, and serve.

PER SERVING: CALORIES: 374 / FAT: 31G / TOTAL CARBS: 8G
FIBER: 3G / NET CARBS: 5G / SUGAR: 3G / PROTEIN: 19G

Fat 75% / Carbs 5% / Protein 20%   Ratio: 2:1

FOR THE DRESSING
⅓ cup extra-virgin olive oil
Juice of 1 lime
2 tablespoons soy sauce
2 teaspoons sambal oelek
1 teaspoon fish sauce
1 (7g) stevia packet

FOR THE SALAD
4 cups shredded
romaine lettuce
½ cup julienned snow peas
½ cup julienned
red bell pepper
¼ cup chopped fresh
cilantro
½ pound chopped
cooked shrimp
½ cup chopped peanuts,
for garnish

IN MENU FOR WEEKS:

TRY INSTEAD: *Sambal oelek is a spicy chile sauce from Southeast Asia. Sambal is Indonesian for a sauce made with green chiles, and* oelek *refers to the technique to make it using a mortar and pestle. If you do not have this potent sauce, you can use sriracha, hot sauce, or sambal terasi.*

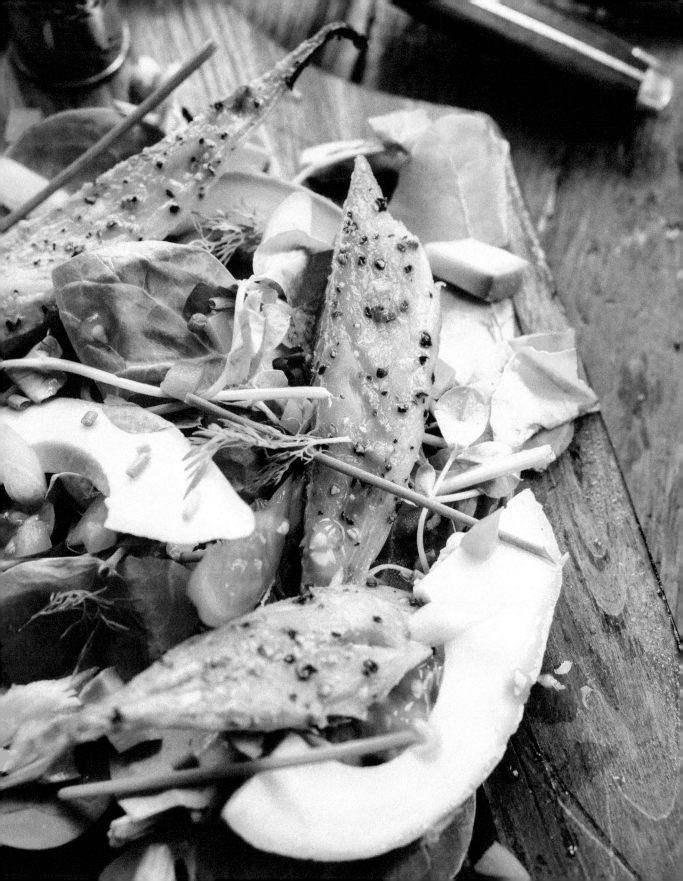

Smoked Trout Salad

SERVES 4 / PREP TIME: 25 MINUTES

Under 30 minutes *Smoked trout is a lovely addition to keto salads because it is high in protein and fat. The fat content in trout is the reason it is a perfect fish for smoking; the fat absorbs the flavor easily. Smoking fish was a preferred method of preserving this food for long ocean voyages and traveling across great distances on land.*

TO MAKE THE DRESSING

1. In a small bowl, whisk together the olive oil, lemon juice, and chives.
2. Season the dressing with salt and pepper, and set aside.

TO MAKE THE SALAD

1. Arrange the watercress, spinach, red pepper, cherry tomatoes, trout, avocado, and dill on 4 plates.
2. Drizzle the dressing over the salads, and serve.

FOR THE DRESSING

½ cup extra-virgin olive oil

¼ cup freshly squeezed lemon juice

1 teaspoon chopped chives

Sea salt

Freshly ground black pepper

FOR THE SALAD

2 cups watercress

2 cups spinach

½ red bell pepper, chopped

½ cup cherry tomatoes, quartered

8 ounces smoked trout

1 avocado, peeled, pitted, and sliced

2 tablespoons chopped dill

PER SERVING: CALORIES: 444 / FAT: 40G / TOTAL CARBS: 5G
FIBER: 3G / NET CARBS: 2G / SUGAR: 1G / PROTEIN: 20G

Fat 78% / Carbs 4% / Protein 18%   Ratio: 2:1

Chicken Caesar Salad

SERVES 4 / PREP TIME: 25 MINUTES

8 cups romaine lettuce

1 cup Traditional Caesar Dressing (page 211)

9 bacon slices, cooked and chopped

½ cup grated Parmesan cheese

1 cup chopped, cooked chicken

Lemon wedges, for garnish

IN MENU FOR WEEKS:

KITCHEN HACK: *Batch cooking can be a convenient method of cutting down the hours you spend in the kitchen on a daily basis. Take some time on the weekend, or a day off, and bake or poach 6 to 10 chicken breasts to use during the week in your recipes. Cooked chicken breasts can be packed into sealed freezer bags and refrigerated for 3 to 4 days or frozen for 1 month.*

Under 30 Minutes • One Pot *Lettuces sometimes seem like they are interchangeable and add bulk more than nutrition to a meal. Romaine lettuce has a distinct crisp, firm texture that is perfect for thick dressings and robust ingredients. It's an exceptional source of vitamin K and very high in vitamins A, B_1, C, and B_2 as well as manganese, potassium, copper, and iron.*

1. In a large bowl, toss the romaine lettuce and Traditional Caesar Dressing together until the lettuce is well coated.

2. Arrange the dressed romaine on 4 plates, and evenly divide the bacon pieces, Parmesan cheese, and chicken over each salad.

3. Serve with lemon wedges.

PER SERVING: CALORIES: 547 / FAT: 45G / TOTAL CARBS: 6G
FIBER: 1G / NET CARBS: 5G / SUGAR: 1G / PROTEIN: 33G

Fat 74% / Carbs 2% / Protein 24%   Ratio: 2:1

Ground Beef Taco Salad

SERVES 4 / PREP TIME: 20 MINUTES / COOK TIME: 6 MINUTES

Under 30 Minutes *The only taco ingredient missing from this salad is the actual corn taco shell that would hold all the seasoned meat, lettuce, cheese, and hot peppers. Eating this combination of ingredients on a plate instead of stuffed into a shell allows you to enjoy the individual components of the dish better. Try a dollop of sour cream as a garnish along with the chopped chipotles.*

1. In a large skillet over medium-high heat, brown the ground beef, stirring frequently, until it is cooked through and browned, about 5 minutes. Pour off any grease, and return the skillet to the heat.

2. Stir in the water and taco seasoning.

3. Cook the meat mixture until the water evaporates, about 1 minute.

4. Remove the skillet from the heat, and set aside.

5. Arrange the lettuce on 4 plates, and top each evenly with the seasoned beef.

6. Evenly divide the avocado, bell pepper, scallion, cheese, cilantro, and jalapeño among the salads.

7. In a small bowl, stir together the Buttermilk Ranch Dressing and chipotle peppers.

8. Spoon the dressing over the salads, and serve.

PER SERVING: CALORIES: 401 / FAT: 31G / TOTAL CARBS: 13G
FIBER: 8G / NET CARBS: 5G / SUGAR: 3G / PROTEIN: 21G

Fat 70% / Carbs 9% / Protein 21%   Ratio: 2:1

½ pound regular ground beef (25% fat)

2 tablespoons water

2 tablespoons taco seasoning

2 cups romaine lettuce

1 avocado, diced

1 green bell pepper, chopped

1 scallion, chopped

½ cup shredded aged Cheddar cheese

¼ cup chopped fresh cilantro

1 jalapeño pepper, thinly sliced

½ cup Buttermilk Ranch Dressing (page 210)

2 chipotle peppers in adobo, chopped

IN MENU FOR WEEKS:

Sirloin Steak Salad
with Goat Cheese and Pecans

SERVES 4 / PREP TIME: 20 MINUTES, PLUS 4 HOURS TO MARINATE / COOK TIME: 10 MINUTES

½ pound sirloin steak

Sea salt

**Freshly ground
black pepper**

**4 tablespoons extra-virgin
olive oil, divided**

**1 teaspoon minced garlic,
divided**

**2 tablespoons apple cider
vinegar**

2 teaspoons Dijon mustard

6 cups spinach

**6 ounces goat cheese,
crumbled**

**¾ cup pecan halves,
toasted**

IN MENU FOR WEEK:

4

TRY INSTEAD: *Goat cheese
can be an acquired taste
for some because it is
characterized by a strong
taste with a "bite" if the
cheese is aged. You can also
use Danish blue, Stilton,
or Roquefort cheese if
you prefer.*

*Picking good-quality beef can be intimidating when confronted by
the extensive selection of confusing cuts available in most grocery
stores. Look for a uniform, clear color (not too bright, which
means it is not aged), and avoid any meat with a slimy surface,
grayish tinge, or dried edges and wet packaging. Buy beef with a
good marbling of fat and even, smooth butchering cuts that follow
the curvature of the muscles.*

1. Season the steak with salt and pepper.

2. Generously rub the steak with 1 tablespoon of olive
   oil and ½ teaspoon of garlic. Refrigerate the steak
   for 3 hours, and let it stand at room temperature for
   45 minutes before grilling it.

3. While the steak is sitting, in a large bowl, whisk together
   the remaining 3 tablespoons of olive oil with the apple
   cider vinegar, Dijon mustard, and remaining ½ teaspoon
   of garlic, and set aside.

4. Preheat a barbecue grill to medium-high or the oven
   to broil.

5. Cook the steak to medium-rare, about 4 minutes per side on the grill or in the oven. Let the steak rest for 10 minutes before slicing it thinly across the grain.

6. Add the spinach to the bowl with the dressing, and toss to coat.

7. Arrange the spinach on 4 plates, and evenly divide the steak among the plates.

8. Top the salads with the goat cheese and pecans, and serve.

PER SERVING: CALORIES: 505 / FAT: 40G / TOTAL CARBS: 5G
FIBER: 2G / NET CARBS: 3G / SUGAR: 2G / PROTEIN: 33G

Fat 71% / Carbs 4% / Protein 26%   Ratio: 2:1

Cauliflower-Cheddar Soup

SERVES 4 / PREP TIME: 10 MINUTES / COOK TIME: 25 MINUTES

8 bacon slices, chopped

1 tablespoon butter

1 sweet onion, chopped

2 teaspoons minced garlic

4 cups cauliflower, chopped into florets

4 cups chicken stock

1 cup heavy (whipping) cream

2 tablespoons water

2 tablespoons arrowroot

1 cup shredded sharp Cheddar cheese, divided

Sea salt

Freshly ground black pepper

A CLOSER LOOK: *Cauliflower is a cruciferous vegetable linked to cancer prevention, detoxification, and heart health. It is packed with antioxidants such as vitamin C and manganese as well as phytonutrients such as beta-carotene. Including cauliflower 2 to 3 times per week in your meals is a good strategy for healthy living.*

Snowy winter days or brisk fall evenings are the best times to curl up with a bowl of this thick, decadent soup. You can certainly enjoy this dish in the spring and summer because cauliflower is available all year, but the peak season is late fall, when large, tightly packed heads of this vegetable taste best. Look for snowy, unblemished heads surrounded by thick, firm leaves to ensure freshness.

1. In a large saucepan over medium-high heat, cook the bacon until crispy, about 5 minutes.

2. Using a slotted spoon, remove the bacon bits and set aside on a plate.

3. Add the butter to the bacon fat in the saucepan, and sauté the onion and garlic until softened, about 3 minutes. Add the cauliflower, and sauté for 1 minute.

4. Stir in the chicken stock, and bring the soup to a boil.

5. Reduce the heat, and simmer until the cauliflower is very tender, about 15 minutes.

6. Transfer the soup to a food processor, add the cream, and purée until very smooth.

7. Return the soup to the saucepan, and place over low heat.

8. In a small bowl, whisk together the water and arrowroot. Whisk the mixture into the soup and ½ cup of the cheese.

9. Stir until the soup thickens, about 2 minutes.

10. Season the soup with salt and pepper.

11. Serve the soup topped with the remaining ½ cup of cheese and reserved bacon bits.

PER SERVING: CALORIES: 386 / FAT: 30G / TOTAL CARBS: 11G
FIBER: 4G / NET CARBS: 7G / SUGAR: 5G / PROTEIN: 20G

Fat 70% / Carbs 9% / Protein 21%   Ratio: 2:1

Watercress-Spinach Soup

SERVES 4 / PREP TIME: 20 MINUTES / COOK TIME: 10 MINUTES

2 tablespoons coconut oil

½ sweet onion, chopped

2 teaspoons minced garlic

1 tablespoon arrowroot

4 cups chicken stock

4 cups watercress

4 cups spinach

1 cup coconut milk

Sea salt

Freshly ground
black pepper

8 cooked turkey bacon
slices, chopped, for garnish

IN MENU FOR WEEK:

1

Under 30 Minutes Watercress is a civilized green that is often used in fine dining as both an ingredient and a lovely garnish. The peppery, subtle taste of this plant is perfect with the more assertive spinach in this gorgeous soup. As its name implies, watercress grows in water, so its freshness is best maintained after purchase by submerging it back in water in a container in the refrigerator.

1. In a large saucepan over medium-high heat, heat the coconut oil.
2. Sauté the onion and garlic in the oil until softened, about 3 minutes.
3. Whisk in the arrowroot to form a paste.
4. Whisk in the chicken stock until the mixture is smooth.
5. Add the watercress, spinach, and coconut milk.
6. Cook the soup until it is just heated through and the greens are still vibrant, about 3 minutes.
7. Transfer the soup to a food processor, and purée.
8. Transfer the soup back to the saucepan, and season with salt and pepper.
9. Top with the bacon, and serve.

PER SERVING: CALORIES: 280 / FAT: 23G / TOTAL CARBS: 7G
FIBER: 4G / NET CARBS: 3G / SUGAR: 3G / PROTEIN: 13G

Fat 74% / Carbs 7% / Protein 19%   Ratio: 2:1

Seafood Chowder

SERVES 4 / PREP TIME: 20 MINUTES / COOK TIME: 20 MINUTES

One Pot *Chowder is historically a peasant food prepared in a large pot or* chaudière, *which is the French word for cauldron. The ingredients of chowder include vegetables and often fish or seafood, depending on the area of the world. You can make this dish with mussels, different types of fish, scallops, and squid.*

1. In a large saucepan over medium-high heat, melt the coconut oil.

2. Sauté the onion, celery, and garlic until softened, about 5 minutes.

3. Stir in the arrowroot, and cook for 2 minutes.

4. Stir in the chicken broth, and cook, stirring constantly, until the soup thickens, about 5 minutes.

5. Stir in the lobster meat, shrimp, cream, and thyme.

6. Cook, stirring occasionally, until the soup is heated through, about 10 minutes. Season the soup with salt and pepper.

7. Top with the chives, and serve.

PER SERVING: CALORIES: 417 / FAT: 32G / TOTAL CARBS: 6G
FIBER: 1G / NET CARBS: 5G / SUGAR: 2G / PROTEIN: 26G

Fat 70% / Carbs 5% / Protein 25%   Ratio: 2:1

4 tablespoons coconut oil

**1 sweet onion,
finely chopped**

**2 celery stalks,
finely chopped**

2 cloves garlic, minced

2 tablespoons arrowroot

3 cups chicken broth

**2 cups cooked, chopped
lobster meat**

**¼ pound cooked shrimp,
chopped**

**1½ cups heavy (whipping)
cream**

**1 teaspoon chopped
fresh thyme**

Sea salt

**Freshly ground
black pepper**

**2 tablespoons chopped
fresh chives**

IN MENU FOR WEEKS:

2   4

Jalapeño-Chicken Soup

SERVES 4 / PREP TIME: 20 MINUTES / COOK TIME: 45 MINUTES

1 tablespoon extra-virgin olive oil

½ pound boneless, skinless chicken thighs, cut into ½-inch pieces

1 sweet onion, diced

2 teaspoons minced garlic

1 carrot, peeled and diced

1 celery stalk, diced

4 jalapeño peppers, diced

1 cup diced tomatoes

2 cups chicken stock

2 teaspoons chili powder

1 teaspoon ground cumin

Pinch ground cayenne pepper

1 cup cream cheese

½ cup heavy (whipping) cream

¼ cup chopped fresh cilantro, for garnish

IN MENU FOR WEEK:

KITCHEN HACK: *Buying a rotisserie chicken at the market and stripping the carcass of meat is a wonderful way to make a couple of meals that require cooked chicken.*

One Pot *This soup might make you sweat, in a healthy way, while you exclaim about the rich, delicious flavor. The peppers add heat, but the addition of chili powder, cumin, and cayenne ensures a complexity that will seem to dance on your taste buds. These spices are combined in many cuisines such as Indian, Indonesian, Asian, and South American. Try grinding whole seeds in a coffee grinder rather than buying a pre-ground product for a fragrant experience.*

1. In a large saucepan over medium-high, heat the olive oil.

2. Brown the chicken thighs until just cooked through, about 10 minutes.

3. Using a slotted spoon, remove the chicken and set aside on a plate.

4. Sauté the onion and garlic until softened, about 3 minutes.

5. Stir in the carrot, celery, jalapeños, tomatoes, chicken stock, chili powder, cumin, cayenne, and the reserved chicken.

6. Bring the soup to a boil, and then reduce the heat to low and simmer the soup until the vegetables are tender, about 30 minutes.

7. Stir in the cream cheese and heavy cream until the cheese is melted.

8. Garnish with the fresh cilantro, and serve.

PER SERVING: CALORIES: 452 / FAT: 35G / TOTAL CARBS: 11G
FIBER: 3G / NET CARBS: 8G / SUGAR: 5G / PROTEIN: 25G

Fat 70% / Carbs 8% / Protein 22%   Ratio: 2:1

Peanut-Chicken Soup

SERVES 4 / PREP TIME: 10 MINUTES / COOK TIME: 15 MINUTES

Under 30 Minutes • One Pot *Peanut soups are popular in West Africa and South America, where they can be as simple as shredded greens in a rich peanut broth or a thick, complex stew with meat, spices, and coconut milk, such as this version. The finished flavor of the soup will depend on the type and amount of curry paste you use. Green curry is quite mild, and if you crave true heat in your soup, try Thai red curry paste.*

1. In a large saucepan over medium-high heat, whisk together the chicken broth, coconut milk, peanut butter, and curry paste.

2. Bring the mixture to a boil, and reduce the heat to simmer for 4 minutes.

3. Stir in the tomatoes, chicken, and garlic powder, and simmer until the mixture is completely heated through, about 5 minutes.

4. Stir in the spinach and cilantro, and simmer until the greens are wilted, about 2 minutes.

5. Remove from the heat, and serve immediately.

2 cups chicken broth

1 cup coconut milk

½ cup natural peanut butter

2 tablespoons curry paste, or more if desired

1 cup diced tomatoes

1 cup shredded cooked chicken breast

1 teaspoon garlic powder

1 cup shredded spinach

1 tablespoon chopped fresh cilantro

IN MENU FOR WEEKS:

PER SERVING: CALORIES: 471 / FAT: 37G / TOTAL CARBS: 14G
FIBER: 5G / NET CARBS: 9G / SUGAR: 5G / PROTEIN: 25G

Fat 71% / Carbs 8% / Protein 21%   Ratio: 2:1

Fiesta Lime Chicken Chowder

SERVES 4 / PREP TIME: 25 MINUTES / COOK TIME: 50 MINUTES

2 tablespoons extra-virgin olive oil

½ pound boneless, skinless chicken thighs, diced

1 sweet onion, chopped

1 jalapeño pepper, diced

2 teaspoons minced garlic

2 cups chicken stock

1 (14-ounce) can diced tomatoes

6 ounces cream cheese

½ cup coconut milk

Juice of 1 lime

2 tablespoons chopped fresh cilantro

½ cup shredded Cheddar cheese, for garnish

IN MENU FOR WEEKS:

 3 4

One Pot *Chicken breast often gets the most attention as the best part of the bird to use in recipes, but the meaty thigh is moister and full of flavor. A comparison between the two chicken parts shows very few nutritional differences. Chicken thighs have slightly less protein and about the same cholesterol, sodium, and iron. A 3-ounce chicken thigh contains 8 grams more fat and 40 more calories than a comparable portion of chicken breast.*

1. In a large saucepan over medium-high heat, heat the olive oil.

2. Cook the chicken thigh until just cooked through, about 10 minutes, and use a slotted spoon to remove the poultry to a plate.

3. Sauté the onion, jalapeño pepper, and garlic until the vegetables are softened, about 4 minutes.

4. Add the chicken stock, diced tomatoes, and reserved chicken to the pot, and bring the liquid to a boil.

5. Reduce the heat to low, and simmer for 30 minutes.

6. Whisk in the cream cheese, coconut milk, lime juice, and cilantro.

7. Cook until the soup is creamy, about 5 minutes.

8. Top with the cheese, and serve.

PER SERVING: CALORIES: 462 / FAT: 36G / TOTAL CARBS: 11G
FIBER: 3G / NET CARBS: 8G / SUGAR: 5G / PROTEIN: 28G

Fat 70% / Carbs 6% / Protein 24%   Ratio: 2:1

Country Pork and "Rice" Soup

SERVES 4 / PREP TIME: 25 MINUTES / COOK TIME: 1 HOUR, 20 MINUTES

One Pot *Thyme is a lovely herb, often used in perennial borders because of its delicate appearance and pungent fragrance. This unassuming little plant has been used for centuries in a medicinal capacity to treat respiratory ailments. Thyme contains several volatile oil components and flavonoids that act as an antimicrobial, antibacterial, and antioxidant in the body.*

1. In a large saucepan over medium-high heat, heat the olive oil.

2. Brown the pork until it is almost cooked through, about 10 minutes.

3. Using a slotted spoon, remove the pork, and set aside.

4. Sauté the onion and garlic until softened, about 3 minutes.

5. Add the pork back to the saucepan, and stir in the chicken stock, coconut milk, tomato, and thyme.

6. Bring the soup to a boil, and then reduce the heat to simmer until the meat is very tender, about 1 hour.

7. Stir in the cauliflower, and simmer the soup until the cauliflower is tender but not overcooked, about 3 minutes.

8. Season the soup with salt and pepper, and serve.

PER SERVING: CALORIES: 410 / FAT: 32G / TOTAL CARBS: 9G
FIBER: 4G / NET CARBS: 5G / SUGAR: 4G / PROTEIN: 25G

Fat 70% / Carbs 5% / Protein 25%   Ratio: 2:1

2 tablespoons extra-virgin olive oil

1 pound boneless country pork ribs, cut into 1-inch pieces

½ sweet onion, chopped

2 teaspoons minced garlic

1 cup chicken stock

1 cup coconut milk

1 large tomato, chopped

1 tablespoon chopped fresh thyme

2 cups finely chopped cauliflower

Sea salt

Freshly ground black pepper

IN MENU FOR WEEKS:

3   4

A CLOSER LOOK: *Pork is leaner than chicken, depending on what cut you use, so try to use the country ribs specified in the recipe to get the correct fat content. Pork is also very high in protein, providing all 9 essential amino acids, and low in natural sodium.*

Beef-Sausage Stew

SERVES 4 / PREP TIME: 30 MINUTES / COOK TIME: 1 HOUR, 30 MINUTES

2 tablespoons extra-virgin olive oil

¼ pound chuck roast, cut into 1-inch pieces

1 sweet onion, chopped

1 teaspoon minced garlic

1½ cups beef broth, divided

½ pound cooked sausage, cut into ¼-inch rounds

3 cups shredded cabbage

½ cup sliced carrots

½ cup peas

1 teaspoon chopped fresh thyme

2 tablespoons arrowroot

Sea salt

Freshly ground black pepper

One Pot *You will not need a great deal of beef to create a hearty stew because the sausage is so rich and the fresh shredded cabbage adds satisfying bulk. If you have a couple of portions of stew left over, try it reheated over Cauliflower "Rice" (page 153) or freeze the extra for another meal. Make sure you cool the stew down completely in the fridge before placing it in the freezer to avoid freezer burn.*

1. In a large saucepan over medium-high heat, heat the olive oil.

2. Brown the beef on all sides, about 5 minutes.

3. Using a slotted spoon, remove the beef to a plate and set aside.

4. Sauté the onion and garlic until the vegetables are softened, about 3 minutes.

5. Return the beef to the saucepan, and add 1¼ cups of beef broth and the sausage.

6. Bring the liquid to a boil, and then reduce the heat to low and simmer, covered, until the beef is very tender, about 1 hour.

7. Stir in the cabbage, carrots, peas, and thyme, and simmer for 15 minutes.

8. In a small bowl, stir together the remaining ¼ cup of beef broth and the arrowroot.

9. Stir the arrowroot mixture into the stew, and stir until the sauce is thickened, about 4 minutes.

10. Season the stew with salt and pepper, and serve.

PER SERVING: CALORIES: 370 / FAT: 27G / TOTAL CARBS: 11G
FIBER: 4G / NET CARBS: 7G / SUGAR: 5G / PROTEIN: 24G

Fat 67% / Carbs 11% / Protein 22%   Ratio: 2:1

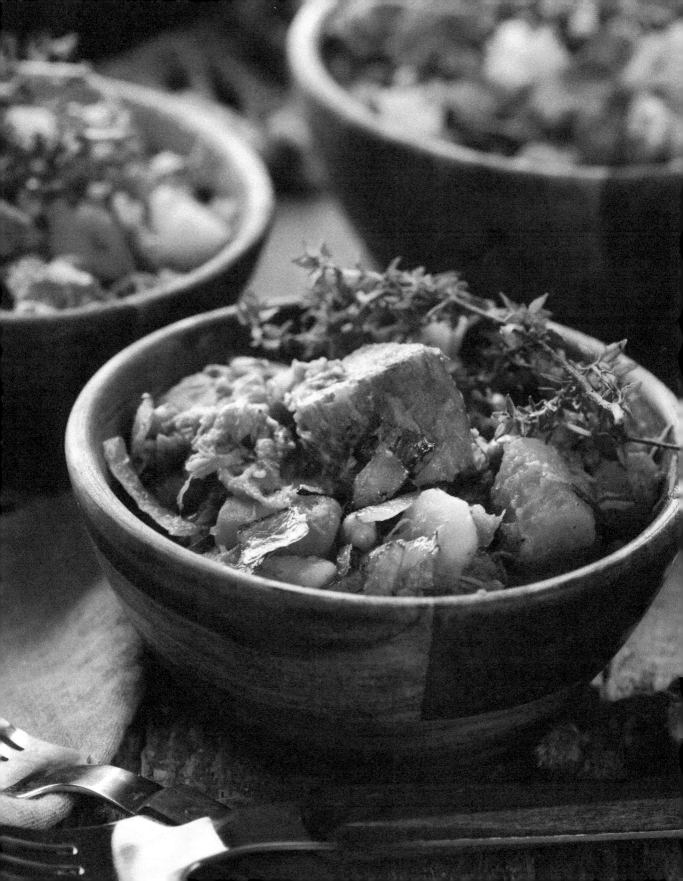

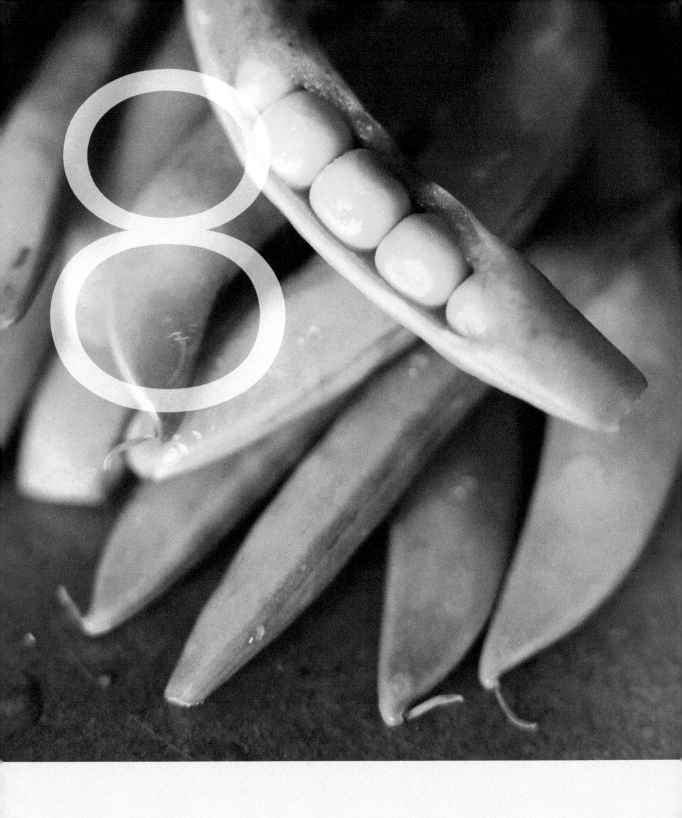

SNACKS

Simple Cheesy Yogurt

SERVES 4 / PREP TIME: 10 MINUTES

¾ cup coconut milk

¾ cup plain Greek yogurt

½ cup cream cheese, softened

¼ teaspoon stevia

TRY INSTEAD: *This yogurt is a very versatile addition to your culinary repertoire because it can serve as a base for many other delectable creations. Try it topped with fresh fruit, stirred into a smoothie or soup, or scooped into a coconut pie crust as a fabulous dessert.*

IN MENU FOR WEEK:

Under 30 Minutes • One Pot • Make Ahead *Greek yogurt is thick and creamy because the whey is strained out, leaving more protein and less carbohydrates. This combination of macronutrients makes the yogurt a fabulous choice for a keto lifestyle. A 6-ounce portion of Greek yogurt has as much protein as a 3-ounce portion of red meat. Read the label on your favorite product to ensure it is real Greek yogurt; you should only see milk and live active cultures.*

1. In a medium bowl, whisk together the coconut milk, Greek yogurt, cream cheese, and stevia until very smooth.
2. Serve.

PER SERVING: CALORIES: 242 / FAT: 22G / TOTAL CARBS: 6G
FIBER: 2G / NET CARBS: 4G / SUGAR: 4G / PROTEIN: 5G

Fat 79% / Carbs 11% / Protein 10%   Ratio: 4:1

Orange Cream Ice Pops

MAKES 8 POPS / PREP TIME: 5 MINUTES, PLUS 3 HOURS TO FREEZE

Make Ahead *Orange and vanilla combine in a luscious, refreshing treat for those days when the temperatures are high and the windows sweat from the humidity. These ice pops do not have the two-tone orange and white of commercially prepared Creamsicles, but the taste is almost identical. Do not substitute orange juice for the extract, or the bright orange flavor will not be as strong.*

1. In a blender, blend the almond milk, cream cheese, egg white protein powder, orange extract, vanilla, stevia, and sea salt until the mixture is very smooth.

2. Pour the mixture into 8 ice pop molds, freeze for at least 3 hours, and serve.

2 cups unsweetened almond milk

¾ cup cream cheese, softened

3 tablespoons egg white protein powder

2 teaspoons orange extract

2 teaspoons pure vanilla extract

½ teaspoon stevia

Pinch sea salt

PER SERVING: CALORIES: 92 / FAT: 8G / TOTAL CARBS: 1G
FIBER: 0G / NET CARBS: 1G / SUGAR: 0G / PROTEIN: 4G

Fat 77% / Carbs 1% / Protein 22%   Ratio: 2:1

Goat Cheese Nuggets

MAKES 16 NUGGETS / PREP TIME: 20 MINUTES, PLUS CHILLING TIME

8 ounces goat cheese

3 oil-packed sun-dried tomatoes

1 teaspoon coconut oil

Pinch red pepper flakes

½ cup walnuts, coarsely ground

A CLOSER LOOK: *Goat cheese has a unique tangy taste and pleasing velvety texture. It is higher in protein, calcium, vitamin A, niacin, and vitamin B6 than cow's milk cheese. Goat cheese is also more digestible, so people who are lactose intolerant can often tolerate it.*

One Pot • Make Ahead *Goat cheese is a forgiving ingredient that can be mixed with many delectable foods to create a scrumptious snack. Hot peppers, olives, artichokes, scallions, mushroom, and other cheeses combine beautifully with creamy goat cheese. You can also swap the walnuts for cashews, pistachios, almonds, and even coconut for a different texture and flavor. If you are having a get-together, create a tray full of unique options for your guests to enjoy.*

1. In a blender, blend the goat cheese, sun-dried tomatoes, coconut oil, and red pepper flakes until well combined.

2. Transfer the cheese mixture to a small bowl, and refrigerate until it is firm enough to roll into balls.

3. Roll the goat cheese mixture into 16 small balls, and roll the balls in the ground walnuts until they are completely coated.

4. Store the goat cheese nuggets in the refrigerator in a sealed container for up to 1 week.

PER SERVING (1 NUGGET): CALORIES: 96 / FAT: 8G / TOTAL CARBS: 1G
FIBER: 0G / NET CARBS: 1G / SUGAR: 0G / PROTEIN: 5G

Fat 75% / Carbs 4% / Protein 21%   Ratio: 2:1

Parmesan Crisps

MAKES 12 CRISPS / PREP TIME: 10 MINUTES / COOK TIME: 5 MINUTES

Under 30 Minutes • One Pot • Make Ahead *Some recipes make you wonder how the dish first came to be, what series of events occurred that resulted in the food on your plate. For example, simple grated cheese mounded on a baking sheet and heated in the oven becomes delicate, lacy, golden crisps that are utterly addictive. You can eat them as a delightful snack or use them as a pretty garnish for Chicken Caesar Salad (page 104) or an entrée. These crisps will last approximately 4 days in a sealed container in the refrigerator.*

¾ cup grated Parmesan cheese

1. Preheat the oven to 400°F.

2. Line a baking sheet with parchment paper.

3. Drop mounds of Parmesan cheese from a tablespoon onto the parchment paper about 1 inch apart.

4. Bake the cheese in the oven until golden, lacy, and crisp, about 5 minutes.

5. Cool and serve.

PER SERVING (2 CRISPS): CALORIES: 47 / FAT: 3G / TOTAL CARBS: 0G
FIBER: 0G / NET CARBS: 0G / SUGAR: 0G / PROTEIN: 5G

Fat 58% / Carbs 10% / Protein 42%   Ratio: 1:2

Cheesy Shrimp Spread

MAKES 1½ CUPS / PREP TIME: 10 MINUTES

6 ounces cream cheese, softened

¼ cup Mayonnaise (page 213)

6 ounces cooked shrimp, chopped

1 tablespoon freshly squeezed lemon juice

1 tablespoon chopped scallion

1 teaspoon chopped fresh dill

Pinch red pepper flakes

Sea salt

Freshly ground black pepper

A CLOSER LOOK: *Shrimp is a low-calorie, high-protein choice for a healthy lifestyle. This tasty shellfish is also high in selenium, vitamin B$_{12}$, and healthy omega-3 fatty acids. Shrimp can reduce the risk of cardiovascular disease and help control blood pressure.*

Under 30 Minutes • One Pot • Make Ahead *You have not had a sublime snacking experience until you've spread this green-flecked pink mixture onto a celery stalk and bitten in. The crisp vegetable, sweet shellfish, and tangy cheese are a sensation in your mouth. The spread can be heated up and served in a pretty ceramic crock as a dip as well, with Nut Crackers (page 130) or cut-up vegetables.*

1. In a food processor, pulse the cream cheese, Mayonnaise, shrimp, lemon juice, scallion, dill, and red pepper flakes until the spread is thick and well blended.

2. Season the spread with salt and pepper.

3. Refrigerate in a sealed container for up to 4 days.

PER SERVING (3 TABLESPOONS): CALORIES: 130 / FAT: 10G
TOTAL CARBS: 3G / FIBER: 0G / NET CARBS: 3G
SUGAR: 1G / PROTEIN: 7G

Fat 70% / Carbs 8% / Protein 22%   Ratio: 2:1

Guacamole

SERVES 8 / PREP TIME: 20 MINUTES

Under 30 Minutes • One Pot • Make Ahead *Guacamole recipes are often family secrets, the subject of heated debates between professional chefs, and the focus of cooking competitions. Chopped or mashed avocado, onion or scallion, garlic or hot peppers, and how much lime juice is needed all are open to debate. This simple recipe has a little heat, a touch of crunch, chunks of buttery avocado, and enough lime juice to ensure that the color stays a lovely green.*

1. In a medium bowl, stir together the avocado, onion, lime juice, egg white protein powder, cilantro, red pepper flakes, and garlic until mixed.

2. Season with salt and pepper, transfer the guacamole to a container, and refrigerate, covered, for up to 2 days.

PER SERVING (¼ CUP): CALORIES: 113 / FAT: 9G / TOTAL CARBS: 6G
FIBER: 4G / NET CARBS: 2G / SUGAR: 1G / PROTEIN: 2G

Fat 72% / Carbs 20% / Protein 8%   Ratio: 4:1

2 avocados, peeled, pitted, and chopped

½ red onion, finely chopped

Juice of 1 lime

1 tablespoon egg white protein powder

2 teaspoons chopped fresh cilantro

1 teaspoon red pepper flakes

1 teaspoon minced garlic

Sea salt

Freshly ground black pepper

Cauliflower Hummus

MAKES 3 CUPS / PREP TIME: 15 MINUTES

3 cups chopped cooked cauliflower

¼ cup freshly squeezed lemon juice

¼ cup extra-virgin olive oil

2 tablespoons tahini paste

2 tablespoons egg white protein powder

1 teaspoon minced garlic

½ teaspoon sea salt

Under 30 Minutes • One Pot • Make Ahead *Traditional nutrient-packed hummus has as its base chickpeas, tahini, lemon juice, and garlic in varying amounts. People often add other ingredients such as olive oil, cilantro, roasted red pepper, and hot peppers. In this case, the chickpeas are swapped out for cauliflower, which has considerably fewer carbs than the original legume. The texture of the cauliflower is quite similar to puréed chickpeas, so see if anyone notices the difference.*

1. In a food processor, pulse the cauliflower, lemon juice, olive oil, tahini, egg white protein powder, garlic, and salt until the hummus is smooth.

2. Transfer the hummus to a sealed container, and refrigerate for up to 1 week.

PER SERVING (¼ CUP): CALORIES: 72 / FAT: 6G / TOTAL CARBS: 2G
FIBER: 1G / NET CARBS: 1G / SUGAR: 1G / PROTEIN: 2G

Fat 75% / Carbs 12% / Protein 13%   Ratio: 3:1

Coconut Tzatziki

SERVES 4 / PREP TIME: 10 MINUTES, PLUS OVERNIGHT TO CHILL

Under 30 Minutes • One Pot • Make Ahead *It might be no surprise to discover that cucumber belongs to the same family as melons, squash, and zucchini when you consider the seeds, shape, and fresh taste of the vegetable. Cucumber is a rich source of phyto-nutrients, vitamin C, and beta-carotene. Cucumber can help fight cancer, detoxify the body, and decrease inflammation. Look for cucumbers in refrigerated sections of your grocery store because this vegetable is sensitive to heat. Try to use the cucumbers you purchase within a couple of days because they lose quality quite quickly.*

1. In a medium bowl, stir together the cucumber, yogurt, coconut milk, garlic, lemon juice, coconut oil, dill, and salt.

2. Refrigerate overnight in a sealed container.

3. Serve.

PER SERVING: CALORIES: 149 / FAT: 12G / TOTAL CARBS: 4G
FIBER: 1G / NET CARBS: 3G / SUGAR: 3G / PROTEIN: 4G

Fat 76% / Carbs 12% / Protein 12%   Ratio: 3:1

1 cup grated cucumber, with the liquid squeezed out

½ cup plain Greek yogurt

½ cup coconut milk

1 teaspoon minced garlic

2 tablespoons freshly squeezed lemon juice

2 tablespoons coconut oil, melted

1 teaspoon chopped fresh dill

Pinch sea salt

KITCHEN HACK: *If you are looking for a fresh-tasting dip, easy topping for burgers or grilled fish, and a fresh salad for a scorching summer day, tzatziki is a perfect choice. This dish gets better after chilling in the fridge and lasts several days, so make a double batch and use it over and over to enhance your meals.*

Feta Cheese Kebabs

SERVES 4 / PREP TIME: 25 MINUTES / COOK TIME: 6 MINUTES

**8 ounces feta cheese,
cut into 12 chunks**

**1 large carrot, cut into
8 ribbons and blanched
until tender crisp**

**1 zucchini,
cut into 12 slices**

**½ red onion,
cut into 8 wedges**

**2 tablespoons extra-virgin
olive oil**

Sea salt

**Freshly ground
black pepper**

**1 tablespoon
black sesame seeds**

Under 30 Minutes • One Pot • Make Ahead *Carrots add a pleasant sweetness and crunch to these kebabs that combine well with the salty feta cheese. This lovely vegetable is full of antioxidants, including hydroxycinnamic acids, anthocyanindins, and beta-carotene, which are powerful disease fighters. Carrots can have a significant impact on the risk of cardiovascular disease, and they promote great vision.*

1. Preheat the oven to broil.
2. Line a baking sheet with aluminum foil, and set the oven rack about 4 inches from the heat.
3. Thread the feta, carrot (doubled over), zucchini, and onion onto 4 metal skewers or onto wood skewers that have been soaked in water for 30 minutes.
4. Brush the kebabs generously with olive oil on all sides, and place them on the baking sheet.
5. Season the kebabs with salt and pepper.
6. Broil the kebabs until the vegetables and cheese are lightly browned, turning to brown all sides, for about 6 minutes in total.
7. Sprinkle with the sesame seeds, and serve immediately.

PER SERVING (1 KEBAB): CALORIES: 243 / FAT: 20G / TOTAL CARBS: 7G
FIBER: 2G / NET CARBS: 5G / SUGAR: 5G / PROTEIN: 10G

Fat 74% / Carbs 10% / Protein 16%   Ratio: 3:1

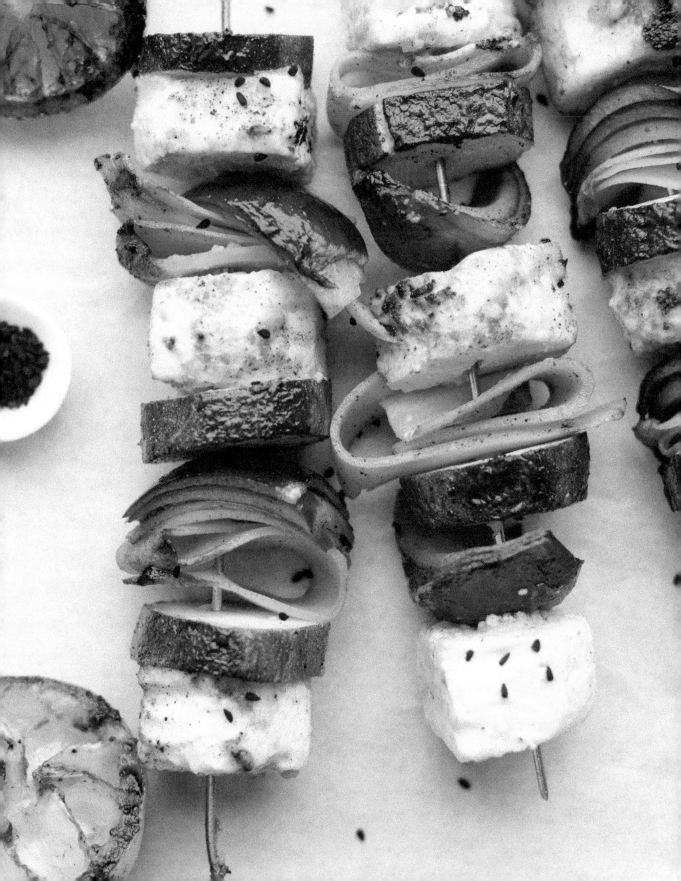

Nut Crackers

SERVES 12 / PREP TIME: 25 MINUTES / COOK TIME: 10 MINUTES

1 cup almond flour

2 tablespoons egg white protein powder

¼ cup ground walnuts

2 tablespoons extra-virgin olive oil

2 egg whites

A CLOSER LOOK: *One ounce of walnuts contains 5 grams of protein and a whopping 18 grams of fat, mostly unsaturated fat. When grinding up the walnuts for this recipe, it is important to leave the whitish waxy skin on the nut because it contains approximately 90% of the phenols in walnuts. Phenols are antioxidants that support good health.*

Make Ahead *It takes very few ingredients to create crunchy, golden crackers that hit the spot when you need a quick pick-me-up. Although the portion size is only two crackers, the calories are low enough that four will not take you over the limit for the day. If you do not care for walnuts because of their slightly bitter taste, pecans can be used instead. Keep in mind that pecans have more fat, carbs, and calories as well as less protein than walnuts if you make the switch.*

1. Preheat the oven to 350°F.
2. Line a 9-by-13-inch baking dish with parchment, and set aside.
3. In a medium bowl, stir together the almond flour, egg white protein powder, and ground walnuts.
4. Stir in the olive oil and egg whites to form a stiff dough.
5. Press the dough evenly into the baking dish, and use a paring knife to cut the dough into 24 squares.
6. Bake until the crackers are golden brown, about 10 minutes.
7. Cool the crackers in the baking dish, and then refrigerate the cooled crackers in a sealed container for up to 1 week.

PER SERVING (2 CRACKERS): CALORIES: 96 / FAT: 8G
TOTAL CARBS: 2G / FIBER: 1G / NET CARBS: 1G
SUGAR: 0G / PROTEIN: 4G

Fat 75% / Carbs 10% / Protein 15%   Ratio: 3:1

Peanut Butter Cookies

MAKES 20 COOKIES / PREP TIME: 10 MINUTES / COOK TIME: 15 MINUTES

Under 30 Minutes • Make Ahead *Xylitol is a sweetener that is a naturally occurring sugar alcohol, and since it looks and tastes like regular granulated sugar, it can be used in the same quantities. This carb is manufactured in the human body, about 15 grams per day through normal metabolism, but as a commercial sweetener, it is processed from products such as corn cobs and hardwood. Xylitol does not raise blood sugar levels or cause tooth decay, but it can create digestive issues in some people and is extremely toxic for dogs, so do not feed your pet these cookies.*

½ cup natural peanut butter

5 tablespoons butter

1 tablespoon heavy (whipping) cream

1 large egg

1½ cups almond flour

½ cup xylitol

¼ cup egg white protein powder

1 teaspoon baking powder

¼ teaspoon baking soda

1. Preheat the oven to 350°F.

2. Line a baking sheet with parchment paper, and set aside.

3. In a large bowl, beat together the peanut butter, butter, cream, and egg until creamy and smooth.

4. Stir in the almond flour, xylitol, egg white protein powder, baking powder, and baking soda.

5. Make 20 balls of dough, and place them on the baking sheet.

6. Press down the balls using a fork to create a cross-hatch design.

7. Bake the cookies until they are crisp and lightly brown, about 15 minutes.

8. Cool the cookies on a wire rack, and refrigerate in a sealed container for up to 1 week.

PER SERVING: CALORIES: 134 / FAT: 11G / TOTAL CARBS: 4G
FIBER: 1G / NET CARBS: 3G / SUGAR: 1G / PROTEIN: 4G

Fat 74% / Carbs 13% / Protein 13%   Ratio: 3:1

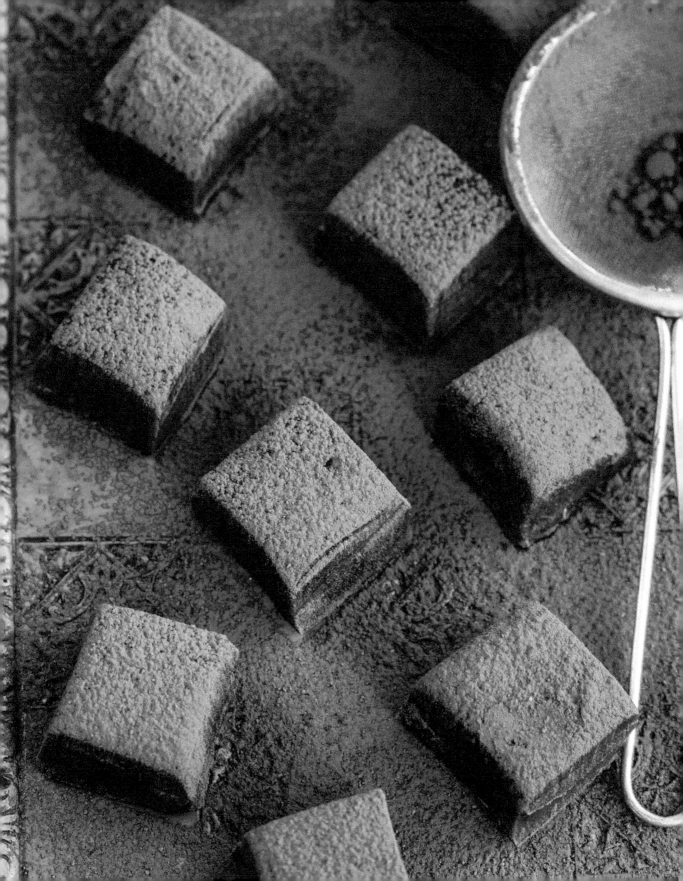

Chocolate Fudge

MAKES 32 PIECES / PREP TIME: 10 MINUTES, PLUS 4 HOURS TO CHILL / COOK TIME: 10 MINUTES

Make Ahead *Good things can come in small packages, and marvelous things can come in a single-piece serving size. Snacks do not have to fill you up or tide you over until the next meal. Snacks can also be a food that relieves a craving or savored slowly because creamy fudgy goodness is exactly what you need in that moment. In order to achieve perfect velvety texture, make sure you whisk the cream cheese and cream until there are absolutely no lumps.*

1. In a large saucepan over medium heat, melt the butter.

2. In a small bowl, whisk the heavy cream and cream cheese until the mixture is very smooth.

3. Add the cream mixture and the stevia to the saucepan, and whisk until smooth.

4. Bring the mixture to a boil, reduce the heat to low, and whisk in the cocoa powder, egg white protein powder, and salt.

5. Simmer for 1 minute, stirring constantly.

6. Pour the chocolate mixture into the baking dish, and refrigerate it to harden, at least 4 hours.

7. Cut the fudge into 32 small squares, and refrigerate in a sealed container for up to 1 week.

PER SERVING (1 PIECE): CALORIES: 75 / FAT: 7G / TOTAL CARBS: 1G
FIBER: 0G / NET CARBS: 1G / SUGAR: 0G / PROTEIN: 2G

Fat 84% / Carbs 5% / Protein 11%   Ratio: 3:1

½ cup butter

1 cup heavy (whipping) cream

12 ounces cream cheese

1 teaspoon stevia

½ cup unsweetened cocoa powder

¼ cup egg white protein powder

Pinch sea salt

A CLOSER LOOK: *Cocoa was a common folk medicine hundreds of years ago, which is no surprise because this powder has significant health benefits. Cocoa is an exceptional source of polyphenolic flavonoids (antioxidants), which can help support a healthy cardiovascular system and lower blood sugar.*

Smoked Salmon Wraps

MAKES 12 WRAPS / PREP TIME: 20 MINUTES

¼ cup cottage cheese

¼ cup cream cheese

1 teaspoon freshly
squeezed lemon juice

2 tablespoons finely
chopped dill

Freshly ground
black pepper

8 smoked Atlantic
salmon strips

Chives, to tie around
the wraps

Under 30 Minutes • Make Ahead *Somewhere, at a picnic or potluck event, there is a plate of delicious smoked salmon wraps waiting to be enjoyed. This dish is a staple hors d'oeuvre, so why not keep some on hand for a quick, tasty snack at home? Smoked salmon is so rich, you will only need two wraps to satisfy any snack cravings. Pacific smoked salmon is a nice substitution, although it can be more expensive. The color of Pacific smoked salmon is a deeper red, and the flavor is often stronger.*

1. In a small bowl, stir together the cottage cheese, cream cheese, lemon juice, and dill until smooth and well blended, about 3 minutes.

2. Season the mixture with pepper.

3. Lay the smoked salmon strips out on a clean work surface, and evenly divide the cheese mixture between them, placing the mixture at the far end of each strip.

4. Roll the first strip toward you, and tie a chive around it to secure the wrap.

5. Repeat with the remaining strips, and serve 2 wraps per person.

6. Refrigerate the wraps, covered, for up to 2 days.

PER SERVING (2 STRIPS): CALORIES: 408 / FAT: 31G / TOTAL CARBS: 6G
FIBER: 0G / NET CARBS: 0G / SUGAR: 0G / PROTEIN: 25G

Fat 71% / Carbs 4% / Protein 25%   Ratio: 1:1

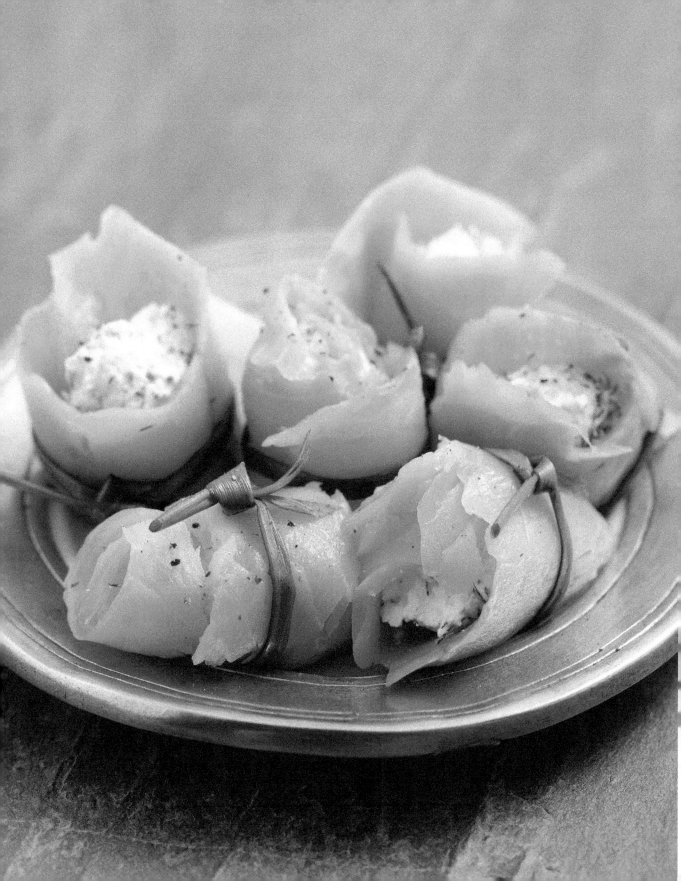

Toasty Granola Bars

MAKES 20 BARS / PREP TIME: 10 MINUTES / COOK TIME: 15 MINUTES

1 cup walnuts

1 cup unsweetened
shredded coconut

1 cup slivered almonds

1 cup roasted
sunflower seeds

¼ cup egg white
protein powder

1 large egg

½ cup natural
peanut butter

¼ cup coconut butter

1 tablespoon
pure vanilla extract

1 teaspoon ground
cinnamon

¼ teaspoon ground nutmeg

Under 30 Minutes • Make Ahead *Commercially manufactured granola bars are not healthy for the most part; they are simply calorie- and sugar-laden cookies packaged in a different shape. People usually grab a granola bar to boost their energy, calm a growling stomach, or even replace a meal, so nutrition is important. The nuts and seeds in this easy homemade bar are packed with healthy fats, protein, vitamins, and minerals. The combination of ingredients is heart friendly and cancer fighting, and it can help control blood sugar.*

1. Preheat the oven to 350°F.

2. In a food processor, pulse the walnuts, coconut, almonds, sunflower seeds, and egg protein powder to coarsely chop the ingredients.

3. Transfer the nut mixture to a large bowl, and stir in the egg, peanut butter, coconut butter, vanilla, cinnamon, and nutmeg until well mixed.

4. Press the granola bar mixture into a 9-by-13-inch baking dish.

5. Using a paring knife, cut the mixture into 24 bars.

6. Bake until the bars are firm and golden, about 15 minutes.

7. Cool the bars in the baking dish, and refrigerate in a sealed container for up to 2 weeks.

PER SERVING: CALORIES: 148 / FAT: 12G / TOTAL CARBS: 4G
FIBER: 2G / NET CARBS: 2G / SUGAR: 1G / PROTEIN: 6G

Fat 73% / Carbs 10% / Protein 17%   Ratio: 2:1

Chicken Salad–Stuffed Avocados

SERVES 4 / PREP TIME: 25 MINUTES

Under 30 Minutes • One Pot *Avocados make a handy, attractive container for this tasty chicken salad filling. Small avocados are best for this snack, or you might find yourself too full for a real meal. If the hollow of the avocado is too shallow after you remove the pit, carefully scoop out a couple spoonfuls of green flesh to create more room. Either mash the removed avocado into the chicken salad or save it for another recipe.*

1. Place the avocado halves on a plate, and set aside.

2. In a medium bowl, stir together the chicken, Mayonnaise, scallion, lemon juice, coconut oil, paprika, garlic powder, and cayenne until well mixed.

3. Spoon the chicken mixture evenly between the avocado halves, sprinkle each with Parmesan cheese, and serve.

PER SERVING: CALORIES: 361 / FAT: 28G / TOTAL CARBS: 12G
FIBER: 7G / NET CARBS: 5G / SUGAR: 2G / PROTEIN: 19G

Fat 70% / Carbs 10% / Protein 20%   Ratio: 2:1

2 small avocados, peeled and pitted

1½ cups chopped cooked chicken

¼ cup Mayonnaise (page 213)

1 tablespoon chopped scallion

1 tablespoon freshly squeezed lemon juice

1 teaspoon coconut oil

½ teaspoon ground paprika

¼ teaspoon garlic powder

¼ teaspoon ground cayenne pepper

2 tablespoons Parmesan cheese

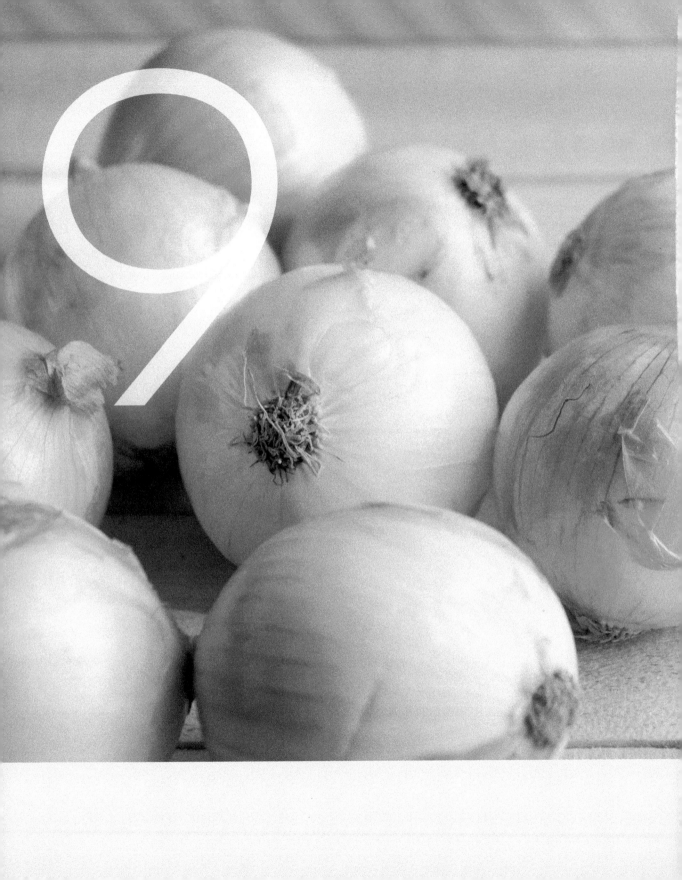

SIDES

Asian Cabbage Stir-Fry

SERVES 4 / PREP TIME: 30 MINUTES / COOK TIME: 15 MINUTES

2 tablespoons sesame oil

1 sweet onion, thinly sliced

2 celery stalks, thinly sliced

1 teaspoon minced garlic

½ red bell pepper,
cut into thin strips

1 cup sliced mushrooms

½ cup cashew halves

¼ cup chicken stock

2 tablespoons soy sauce

½ pound finely shredded
green cabbage

1 tablespoon sesame seeds

One Pot *Adding a little chopped chicken, pork, or whole shrimp to this recipe can quickly turn this fragrant side dish into a satisfying main course. You can also eat any leftovers cold because the lightly flavored vegetables stay tender-crisp in the refrigerator, and the flavor is even better the second day. You can substitute any keto lifestyle–friendly vegetables with good results, such as snow peas, asparagus, carrots, green beans, and broccoli.*

1. In a large skillet over medium heat, heat the sesame oil.

2. Sauté the onion, celery, and garlic until softened, about 5 minutes.

3. Add the red pepper, mushrooms, and cashews, and stir-fry for 3 minutes.

4. Stir in the chicken stock, soy sauce, and cabbage.

5. Cover the skillet, and steam the cabbage until it is tender, about 5 minutes.

6. Top with the sesame seeds, and serve.

PER SERVING: CALORIES: 151 / FAT: 12G / TOTAL CARBS: 10G
FIBER: 4G / NET CARBS: 6G / SUGAR: 4G / PROTEIN: 4G

Fat 72% / Carbs 18% / Protein 10%   Ratio: 3:1

Sesame-Roasted Broccoli

SERVES 4 / PREP TIME: 5 MINUTES / COOK TIME: 10 MINUTES

Under 30 Minutes *Broccoli should be included at least 2 to 3 times per week in your meals because it has an incredibly positive impact on your health. Broccoli can lower cholesterol levels, reduce body-wide inflammation, support the digestive and cardiovascular systems, and help detox your body. Broccoli is exceptionally high in vitamins K and C as well as rich in chromium, vitamin E, phosphorous, and manganese.*

1. Preheat the oven to 425°F.
2. Lightly oil a baking sheet with olive oil.
3. In a large bowl, toss the broccoli florets with the sesame oil and garlic.
4. Transfer the broccoli to the baking sheet, and spread it out in a single layer.
5. Roast the broccoli until tender, about 10 minutes.
6. Transfer the roasted broccoli to a serving bowl, top with the lemon juice and sesame seeds, and serve.

PER SERVING: CALORIES: 131 / FAT: 11G / TOTAL CARBS: 6G
FIBER: 3G / NET CARBS: 3G / SUGAR: 2G / PROTEIN: 3G

Fat 75% / Carbs 18% / Protein 7%   Ratio: 3:1

Extra-virgin olive oil, for greasing

4 cups broccoli, cut into small florets

3 tablespoons sesame oil

1 teaspoon garlic

1 teaspoon freshly squeezed lemon juice

2 teaspoons sesame seeds

IN MENU FOR WEEK:

1

A CLOSER LOOK: *Sesame oil is one of the healthiest oils in the world and is used medicinally in many countries. Sesame oil can help lower blood sugar, improve oral health, reduce blood pressure, and help cut the risk of heart disease and cancer. Sesame oil is also rancid-resistant, so you can stock up when it is on sale at the supermarket.*

Sautéed Swiss Chard

SERVES 4 / PREP TIME: 15 MINUTES / COOK TIME: 25 MINUTES

6 bacon slices, chopped

2 tablespoons butter

2 tablespoons chopped sweet onion

1 teaspoon minced garlic

8 cups Swiss chard

Sea salt

One Pot *Swiss chard is one of the prettiest greens you can use, with many varieties sporting deep red or yellow stems and coordinated coloring in the veins on the leaves. It is best to only eat the stems of white chard, because the colored stems can be woody and unpalatable. Chard is a close second behind spinach as one of the healthiest vegetables in the world, so you should try to include it in several meals per week.*

1. In a large skillet over medium heat, cook the bacon until crispy, about 5 minutes.
2. Add the butter to the skillet, and melt.
3. Sauté the onion and garlic until the vegetables are softened, about 3 minutes.
4. Stir in the chard, and sauté, stirring occasionally, until the greens wilt, about 20 minutes.
5. Season with salt, and serve.

PER SERVING: CALORIES: 102 / FAT: 8G / TOTAL CARBS: 4G
FIBER: 2G / NET CARBS: 2G / SUGAR: 1G / PROTEIN: 5G

Fat 71% / Carbs 9% / Protein 20%   Ratio: 2:1

Twice-Baked Spaghetti Squash

SERVES 4 / PREP TIME: 20 MINUTES / COOK TIME: 55 MINUTES

Make Ahead *Spaghetti squash is a popular choice for people avoiding grain products because when cooked, the flesh falls away in ribbons that resemble strands of pasta. The flesh can range from creamy white to a deep orange and tastes similar to pumpkin. Spaghetti squash is low in calories and high in beta-carotene, potassium, folic acid, and vitamins A and C, and also contains omega-3 fatty acids, which can help reduce inflammation in the body.*

1. Preheat the oven to 350°F.

2. Line a baking sheet with parchment paper.

3. Lightly drizzle the cut sides of the squash with olive oil, and place them cut-side down on the baking sheet.

4. Bake the squash until it is very tender, about 35 minutes.

5. Scoop the cooked squash flesh into a large bowl, and discard the rinds.

6. Stir in the cream, pancetta, butter, garlic, and scallion.

7. Season the squash mixture with salt and pepper.

8. Spoon the squash mixture into 4 (6-ounce) ramekins.

9. Top each ramekin with ¼ cup of cheese.

10. Bake the squash for 20 minutes, until the Cheddar on top is melted and bubbly, and serve.

PER SERVING: CALORIES: 229 / FAT: 18G / TOTAL CARBS: 6G
FIBER: 0G / NET CARBS: 6G / SUGAR: 0G / PROTEIN: 12G

Fat 71% / Carbs 8% / Protein 21%   Ratio: 2:1

Extra-virgin olive oil, for drizzling

1 spaghetti squash, halved

½ cup heavy (whipping) cream

6 slices cooked pancetta, chopped

2 tablespoons butter

1 teaspoon minced garlic

1 scallion, chopped

Sea salt

Freshly ground black pepper

1 cup shredded Cheddar cheese, divided

IN MENU FOR WEEKS:

KITCHEN HACK: *This entire dish can be made ahead and refrigerated for up to 2 days. Then, simply pull them out, pop them in the oven, and bake. Just increase the cooking time by about 10 minutes if they are completely chilled.*

Zucchini Fritters

SERVES 4 / PREP TIME: 15 MINUTES / COOK TIME: 10 MINUTES

1½ pounds zucchini, grated and the liquid squeezed out

6 tablespoons Parmesan cheese

¼ cup almond flour

1 teaspoon minced garlic

1 large egg, beaten

Dash freshly ground black pepper

2 tablespoons extra-virgin olive oil

IN MENU FOR WEEK:

2

A CLOSER LOOK: *Zucchini, also called a courgette, is a fruit but often prepared as a vegetable. Zucchini is a great source of beta-carotene, protein, potassium, and vitamins A and C. This mild-tasting squash is a mild diuretic and can stimulate the intestines, which supports digestive health.*

Under 30 Minutes *Fritter derives from the Latin word* frictura, *meaning "a fry." Most fritters consist of batter-encased fruit, vegetables, and meat immersed in oil to create a crisp, golden-brown finish. These zucchini fritters are not batter encased, but they still fry up crunchy and delectable. The trick to firm fritters that stay together in the skillet is to completely squeeze out the liquid from the grated zucchini.*

1. In a large bowl, stir together the zucchini, Parmesan cheese, almond flour, garlic, egg, and pepper. Roll the mixture into 12 equal balls, flattening them out slightly.

2. In a large skillet over medium-high heat, heat the olive oil.

3. When the olive oil is sizzling, place 6 zucchini fritters in the skillet, and cook until the bottom is golden brown, about 3 minutes.

4. Turn the fritters over, and brown the other side, about 2 minutes.

5. Transfer the fritters to paper towels, and repeat with the remaining fritters.

6. Serve.

PER SERVING: CALORIES: 187 / FAT: 15G / TOTAL CARBS: 7G
FIBER: 3G / NET CARBS: 4G / SUGAR: 3G / PROTEIN: 8G

Fat 72% / Carbs 8% / Protein 20%   Ratio: 2:1

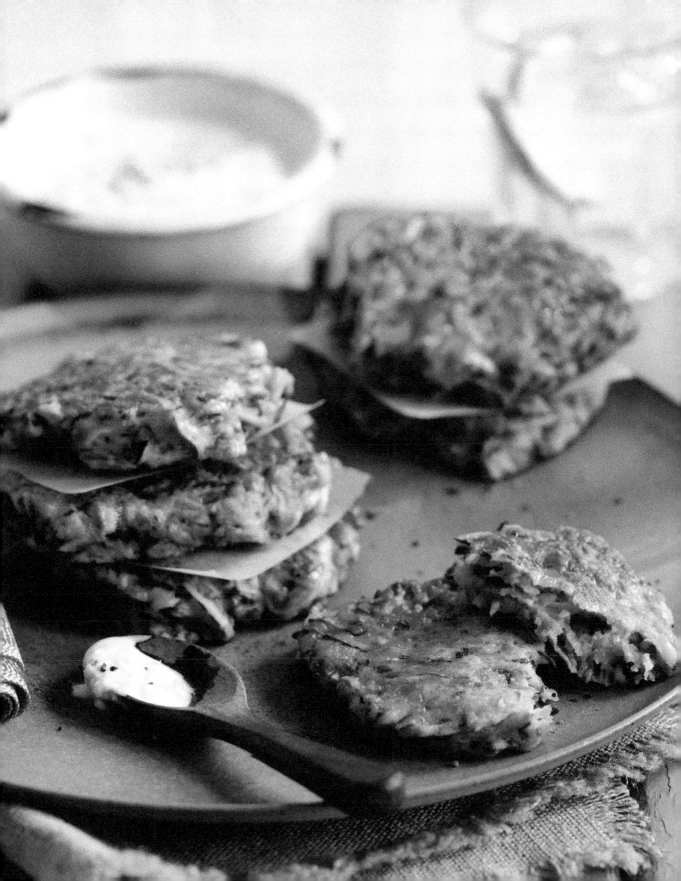

Broccoli-Cauliflower Casserole

SERVES 4 / PREP TIME: 20 MINUTES / COOK TIME: 30 MINUTES

3 cups broccoli florets

3 cups cauliflower florets

1 cup cream cheese

2 tablespoons coconut oil, melted

1 teaspoon minced garlic

¾ cup diced lean ham

½ cup shredded Cheddar cheese

IN MENU FOR WEEKS:

Make Ahead *Casseroles are incredible time savers because you can prepare the entire dish ahead, even the day before, and not have to deal with cleanup on the day you serve it. The addition of ham adds a rich flavor component and protein to the finished dish, but you can omit it. The best ham to eat does not contain high levels of sodium or cancer-causing nitrates, so read the labels carefully to ensure you get a superior product.*

1. Preheat the oven to 400°F.
2. Place a large saucepan filled with water on high heat, and bring the water to a boil.
3. Lightly blanch the broccoli and cauliflower until tender-crisp, about 3 minutes.
4. Drain the vegetables, and transfer them to a large bowl.
5. In a small bowl, whisk together the cream cheese, coconut oil, garlic, and ham.
6. Stir the cream cheese mixture into the broccoli and cauliflower until the vegetables are well coated.
7. Spoon the mixture into an 8-cup casserole dish, and top with the Cheddar cheese.
8. Bake the casserole until heated through, about 20 minutes, and serve.

PER SERVING: CALORIES: 388 / FAT: 32G / TOTAL CARBS: 10G
FIBER: 4G / NET CARBS: 6G / SUGAR: 3G / PROTEIN: 18G

Fat 74% / Carbs 7% / Protein 19%   Ratio: 2:1

Buttery Mashed Cauliflower

SERVES 4 / PREP TIME: 15 MINUTES / COOK TIME: 10 MINUTES

Under 30 Minutes *Mashed potatoes is the most popular side dish in North America by a substantial margin, so finding a comparable side that suits a low-carbohydrate diet is a triumph. Cauliflower purées to a fluffy, thick texture, which is further enhanced by creamy Greek yogurt and pools of melted golden butter. Use any leftover cauliflower mash as a topping on shepherd's pie or as a delicious snack.*

1. In a large saucepan over high heat, bring 3 inches of water to a boil.

2. Place the cauliflower and garlic in a steamer basket or sieve over the water, and steam until the vegetables are very tender, about 10 minutes.

3. Transfer the cauliflower and garlic to a food processor, and add the yogurt, olive oil, 1 tablespoon of butter, and the salt.

4. Purée until the cauliflower is very fluffy, about 2 minutes.

5. Transfer the cauliflower to a serving dish, dot with the remaining 1 tablespoon of butter, and serve.

PER SERVING: CALORIES: 168 / FAT: 13G / TOTAL CARBS: 11G
FIBER: 6G / NET CARBS: 5G / SUGAR: 5G / PROTEIN: 6G

Fat 70% / Carbs 19% / Protein 11%   Ratio: 2:1

8 cups cauliflower

2 teaspoons minced garlic

¼ cup Greek yogurt

2 tablespoons extra-virgin olive oil, divided

2 tablespoons butter, divided

½ teaspoon sea salt

IN MENU FOR WEEKS:

TRY INSTEAD: *The texture of this dish is so close to regular mashed potatoes that you can jazz them up with traditional variations such as roasted garlic, bacon, cheese, and buttermilk. For a more exotic side dish, stir in caviar, grated truffles, or horseradish.*

Creamed Spinach

SERVES 4 / PREP TIME: 5 MINUTES / COOK TIME: 15 MINUTES

1 cup coconut milk

8 cups packed spinach

¼ teaspoon sea salt

1 teaspoon lemon zest

3 tablespoons chopped walnuts

IN MENU FOR WEEKS:

Under 30 Minutes • One Pot *Creamed vegetables seem somehow old-fashioned and comforting, because this cooking technique lost popularity when low-fat diets became all the rage in the 1980s. This version uses coconut milk instead of heavy cream, but the technique is the same. Creamed spinach is best served alongside a hearty entrée such as roast beef, grilled lamb chops, or chicken.*

1. In a large skillet over medium heat, bring the coconut milk to a simmer.
2. Stir in the spinach, salt, and lemon zest. Simmer until the mixture is creamy and the spinach is tender, about 15 minutes.
3. Top with the chopped walnuts, and serve.

PER SERVING: CALORIES: 206 / FAT: 18G / TOTAL CARBS: 6G
FIBER: 3G / NET CARBS: 3G / SUGAR: 2G / PROTEIN: 5G

Fat 78% / Carbs 12% / Protein 10%   Ratio: 2:1

Roasted Asparagus with Goat Cheese

SERVES 4 / PREP TIME: 15 MINUTES / COOK TIME: 15 MINUTES

Under 30 Minutes *Slender, elegant asparagus are surprisingly durable when barbecued, and this dish adds both flavor and disease-fighting antioxidants to your meal. Asparagus is a fabulous source of vitamins A, C, and K as well as many B vitamins. This vegetable can help reduce the risk of cataracts and blindness due to degenerative diseases while promoting a healthy cardiovascular system.*

1. Preheat the oven to 425°F.
2. In a small saucepan over medium heat, heat the olive oil. Heat the garlic, lemon juice, and lemon zest in the oil until the garlic is lightly caramelized, about 5 minutes.
3. In a large bowl, pour the olive oil mixture over the asparagus, and toss to coat.
4. Arrange the olive oil on a baking sheet, and sprinkle the goat cheese evenly over the vegetables.
5. Roast the asparagus in the oven until tender, about 10 minutes, and serve.

¼ cup extra-virgin olive oil

2 teaspoons minced garlic

Juice and zest of ½ lemon

2 pounds asparagus, trimmed

1 cup goat cheese, crumbled

IN MENU FOR WEEKS:

PER SERVING: CALORIES: 284 / FAT: 23G / TOTAL CARBS: 19G
FIBER: 5G / NET CARBS: 5G / SUGAR: 5G / PROTEIN: 14G

Fat 73% / Carbs 7% / Protein 20%   Ratio: 2:1

Spinach Soufflé

SERVES 6 / PREP TIME: 15 MINUTES / COOK TIME: 40 MINUTES

¼ cup butter, softened, plus more for greasing

8 cups spinach, chopped

16 ounces cottage cheese

8 ounces aged Cheddar cheese, cubed

6 eggs, beaten

2 tablespoons almond flour

½ teaspoon sea salt

½ teaspoon ground nutmeg

IN MENU FOR WEEKS:

Make Ahead *Soufflés are one of the trickiest dishes to create, and even professional chefs consider themselves fortunate if theirs don't deflate after removing the dish from the oven. Never fear; this soufflé is not a traditional one, so it will not fall down or require careful supervision and folding of the egg whites. The only precaution to take when making this recipe is to thoroughly squeeze the water from the spinach.*

1. Preheat the oven to 350°F.

2. Lightly grease a 9-by-13-inch casserole dish with butter. Set aside.

3. Place a large saucepan filled with water over high heat, and bring the water to a boil.

4. Blanch the spinach until it is tender, about 2 minutes.

5. Drain the spinach, and squeeze out all the water.

6. Transfer the spinach to a large bowl, and stir in the cottage cheese, Cheddar cheese, eggs, butter, almond flour, salt, and nutmeg.

7. Spoon the mixture into the casserole dish, and bake until the soufflé is set and golden brown, about 35 minutes.

8. Serve.

PER SERVING: CALORIES: 356 / FAT: 28G / TOTAL CARBS: 4G
FIBER: 1G / NET CARBS: 3G / SUGAR: 1G / PROTEIN: 23G

Fat 71% / Carbs 4% / Protein 25%   Ratio: 1:1

Roasted Onions

SERVES 4 / PREP TIME: 15 MINUTES / COOK TIME: 40 MINUTES

Make Ahead *You might want to make a double batch of roasted onions after you taste the surprisingly sweet finished product. A touch of garlic and a smattering of chopped fresh thyme are pleasing additions if you feel the recipe needs a bit of jazzing up. If you happen to have any leftovers, you can use them as a topping on grilled steaks or a delectable omelet filling.*

1. Preheat the oven to 375°F.

2. Lightly grease a baking sheet with olive oil, and arrange the onion slices on the sheet.

3. Drizzle the onion slices with the olive oil, and season with salt and pepper.

4. Roast the onions until golden, about 15 minutes.

5. While the onions are roasting, in a small saucepan over medium-high heat, whisk together the cream and apple cider vinegar.

6. Bring the cream mixture to a simmer, and then remove the saucepan from the heat.

7. Remove the onions from the oven, and increase the oven temperature to 450°F.

8. Transfer the onion to a 9-by-13-inch baking dish, and pour the cream mixture over them.

9. Sprinkle the blue cheese over the onion mixture, and cover the baking dish with foil.

10. Bake the onions in the oven for 15 minutes, remove the foil, and bake for another 10 minutes.

11. Serve.

1 tablespoon extra-virgin olive oil, plus more for greasing

4 sweet onions, cut into ¼-inch slices

Sea salt

Freshly ground black pepper

1 cup heavy (whipping) cream

1 teaspoon apple cider vinegar

¾ cup blue cheese

TRY INSTEAD: *Onions are not all created equal. Different types of these alliums have unique flavors, sugar content, and colors. You can try roasting white onions, but the flavor will not be as rich, and red onions impart a strange pink color to the sauce. Both will work in a pinch, if sweet yellow onions are not available.*

PER SERVING: CALORIES: 267 / FAT: 22G / TOTAL CARBS: 11G
FIBER: 3G / NET CARBS: 8G / SUGAR: 4G / PROTEIN: 7G

Fat 74% / Carbs 16% / Protein 10%   Ratio: 3:1

Nutty Miso "Rice"

SERVES 4 / PREP TIME: 15 MINUTES / COOK TIME: 7 MINUTES

3 cups cauliflower

1 cup fennel

¼ cup walnuts

1 tablespoon extra-virgin olive oil

2 teaspoons white miso

1 teaspoon freshly squeezed lemon juice

Under 30 Minutes *Miso-flavored rice enhances fish dishes exquisitely, especially if the protein is grilled or broiled. You can certainly serve this rice with chicken, pork, or red meat, but the lemony anise taste of the dish seems delicate and easily overpowered. Cashews and pistachios can be used instead of walnuts, and for an interesting variation, try pine nuts for their buttery, slightly resinous flavor.*

1. In a food processor, pulse the cauliflower, fennel, and walnuts until the mixture resembles coarse crumbs.

2. In a large skillet over medium heat, heat the olive oil.

3. Sauté the cauliflower mixture in the oil until heated through and tender, about 6 minutes.

4. Stir in the miso and lemon juice, and sauté for 1 minute.

5. Remove the "rice" from the heat, and serve.

PER SERVING: CALORIES: 167 / FAT: 14G / TOTAL CARBS: 8G
FIBER: 5G / NET CARBS: 3G / SUGAR: 3G / PROTEIN: 5G

Fat 75% / Carbs 14% / Protein 11%   Ratio: 3:1

Cauliflower "Rice"

SERVES 4 / PREP TIME: 15 MINUTES / COOK TIME: 5 MINUTES

Under 30 Minutes • Make Ahead *Rice is a staple food all over the world, both as a side dish and as the main source of carbohydrates. The keto lifestyle does not recommend eating rice, so cauliflower "rice" takes its place in many households following it. Chopped, cooked cauliflower has an almost identical texture to cooked basmati rice. You must watch the cooking time carefully because overcooking the cauliflower will leave you with a mushy mess. If you overcook the cauliflower, mash it up instead with cream and a dollop of butter for mashed "potatoes."*

1. In a food processor, pulse the cauliflower until finely chopped.

2. In a large skillet over medium heat, heat the olive oil.

3. Sauté the garlic until fragrant and softened, about 2 minutes.

4. Add the cauliflower and water to the skillet.

5. Cover the skillet, and steam the cauliflower until tender-crisp, about 2 minutes.

6. Transfer the cauliflower to a bowl, and serve.

PER SERVING: CALORIES: 65 / FAT: 5G / TOTAL CARBS: 5G
FIBER: 3G / NET CARBS: 3G / SUGAR: 3G / PROTEIN: 3G

Fat 70% / Carbs 24% / Protein 6%   Ratio: 2:1

5 cups chopped cauliflower

2 teaspoons extra-virgin olive oil

1 teaspoon minced garlic

2 tablespoons water

IN MENU FOR WEEKS:

TRY INSTEAD: *This quick, mild-tasting dish has a similar texture to real rice, and the mild flavor lends itself well to interesting recipe additions. You can add vegetables, chopped meats, spices, soy sauce, salsa, chopped nuts, fresh herbs, or hot spices to the basic cauliflower "rice" dish, depending on your palate and culinary needs.*

Brussels Sprouts with Hazelnuts

SERVES 4 / PREP TIME: 15 MINUTES / COOK TIME: 15 MINUTES

¾ pound Brussels sprouts, trimmed and halved lengthwise

4 teaspoons coconut oil, melted

½ teaspoon ground coriander

½ cup chopped hazelnuts

IN MENU FOR WEEK:

1

Brussels sprouts, despite their impressive nutritional profile, are not a popular vegetable with many people. The issue usually lies with the unpleasant sulfur smell associated with this cruciferous vegetable. Overcooking Brussels sprouts produces this nasty scent, so make sure they are still tender-crisp when you serve them, and cut them into smaller pieces beforehand so that the cooking time will be reduced.

1. Preheat the oven to 400°F.
2. Line a baking sheet with parchment paper.
3. In a large bowl, toss the Brussels sprouts with the coconut oil and coriander until well coated.
4. Spread the Brussels sprouts on a baking sheet, and bake until tender-crisp, about 15 minutes.
5. Remove the Brussels sprouts from the oven, toss with the chopped hazelnuts, and serve.

PER SERVING: CALORIES: 162 / FAT: 13G / TOTAL CARBS: 9G
FIBER: 5G / NET CARBS: 5G / SUGAR: 2G / PROTEIN: 6G

Fat 69% / Carbs 20% / Protein 11%   Ratio: 2:1

Garlic Green Beans

SERVES 4 / PREP TIME: 15 MINUTES / COOK TIME: 10 MINUTES

Under 30 Minutes *Do not make these beans too long before dinner, or you might find yourself without a side dish for the meal because you will eat them yourself right out of the skillet. Green beans are an excellent source of vitamins B₂, C, and K as well as manganese, copper, iron, and phosphorus. They support a healthy cardiovascular system, help reduce the risk of type 2 diabetes, and reduce inflammation.*

1. Bring a large pot of water to a boil over high heat.

2. Add the beans, cover and cook for 5 to 6 minutes, or until tender-crisp.

3. Drain, and keep warm.

4. In a large skillet over medium heat, heat the coconut oil, and sauté the garlic until softened, about 2 minutes.

5. Add the beans, and toss to coat.

6. Top with walnuts, and serve.

1½ pounds fresh green beans, trimmed

2 tablespoons coconut oil

3 teaspoons minced garlic

4 tablespoons chopped walnuts

KITCHEN HACK: *Finding fresh green beans is not difficult, especially if you live in the United States, where over 60% of the world's green bean crops are found. However, if the quality of fresh products is lacking, you can replace fresh with flash frozen and retain 90% of the vitamins and nutrients.*

PER SERVING: CALORIES: 163 / FAT: 12G / TOTAL CARBS: 13G
FIBER: 7G / NET CARBS: 5G / SUGAR: 3G / PROTEIN: 5G

Fat 72% / Carbs 12% / Protein 16%   Ratio: 2:1

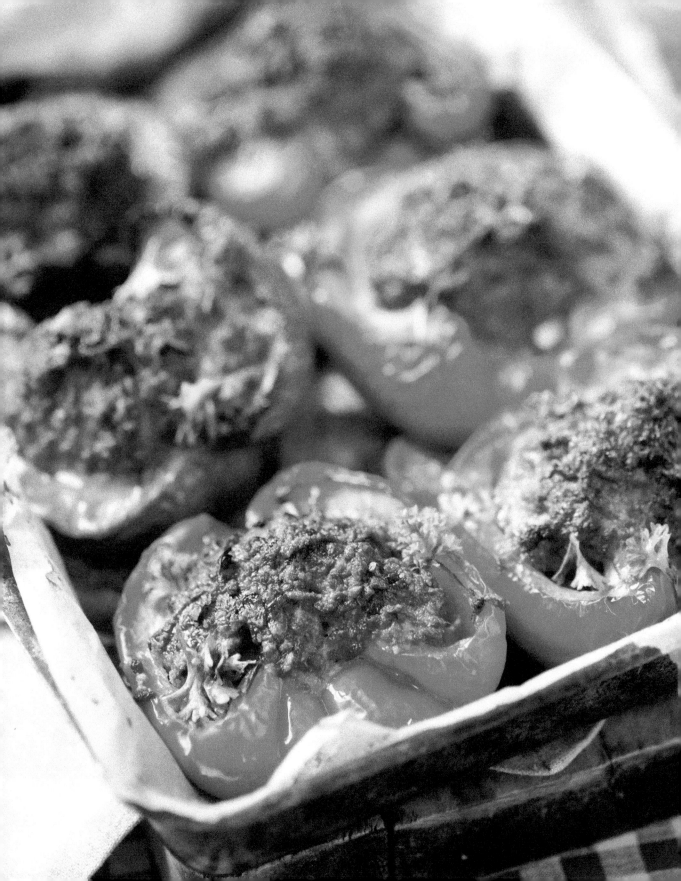

Beef-Stuffed Red Peppers

SERVES 4 / PREP TIME: 20 MINUTES / COOK TIME: 30 MINUTES

Make Ahead *Oregano is one of the herbs used prominently in Greek cuisine, so it is right at home with olive oil and balsamic vinegar. This fragrant herb's name means "mountain joy," which seems fitting because it grows wild as a perennial on hillsides in Mediterranean countries. Oregano is a potent antibacterial and antioxidant as well as a good source of vitamin K, manganese, iron, and calcium. Whenever possible, use fresh oregano in your recipes for a superior flavor, and store the herb wrapped in a paper towel in the refrigerator.*

1. Preheat the oven to 350°F.
2. Rub the red peppers all over generously with the olive oil, and place them open-side up in a 9-by-13-inch baking dish.
3. In a medium bowl, stir together the beef, Parmesan, onion, oregano, garlic, basil, and thyme until well mixed.
4. Evenly divide the meat mixture among the four red peppers, spooning it into the hollows.
5. Cover with foil, and bake the stuffed red peppers until the meat mixture is cooked through and the peppers are tender, about 30 minutes.
6. Serve.

4 red bell peppers, tops cut off and seeded

2 tablespoons extra-virgin olive oil

½ pound ground beef (25% fat)

2 ounces grated Parmesan cheese

½ sweet onion, minced

2 teaspoons chopped fresh oregano

1 teaspoon minced garlic

1 teaspoon chopped fresh basil

¼ teaspoon chopped fresh thyme

PER SERVING: CALORIES: 308 / FAT: 22G / TOTAL CARBS: 8G
FIBER: 3G / NET CARBS: 5G / SUGAR: 5G / PROTEIN: 20G

Fat 64% / Carbs 11% / Protein 25%   Ratio: 2:1

Coconut-Zucchini Noodles

SERVES 4 / PREP TIME: 15 MINUTES

½ avocado, diced

2 tablespoons water

1 tablespoon freshly squeezed lemon juice

1 tablespoon coconut oil

2 tablespoons shredded unsweetened coconut

1 tablespoon chopped cilantro

3 zucchini, cut into long ribbons with a peeler or spiralized

Juice of 1 lime

1 cup blanched asparagus, cut into 2-inch pieces

IN MENU FOR WEEKS:

 2   4

Under 30 Minutes • Make Ahead *If you enjoy creating dishes with lovely presentation, a spiralizer is a handy tool to invest in for recipes such as this one. A spiralizer creates long, uniform vegetable noodles that look fabulous and can substitute for pasta. Spiralizers can be expensive or only a few dollars, depending on whether you mind cranking the noodles out by hand or want to simply press a button.*

1. In a blender, blend the avocado, water, lemon juice, and coconut oil until smooth.

2. Pour the avocado mixture into a bowl, and whisk in the coconut and cilantro. Set aside.

3. In a large bowl, toss the zucchini, lime juice, and asparagus together.

4. Add the sauce, toss to combine well, and serve.

PER SERVING: CALORIES: 131 / FAT: 9G / TOTAL CARBS: 10G
FIBER: 6G / NET CARBS: 4G / SUGAR: 1G / PROTEIN: 5G

Fat 75% / Carbs 16% / Protein 9%   Ratio: 2:1

Whole Roasted Cauliflower

SERVES 6 / PREP TIME: 15 MINUTES / COOK TIME: 30 MINUTES

Hard cheeses often seem interchangeable, but taking the time to source out real Parmesan cheese is worth the effort. In order to be considered a true Parmesan cheese, it has to be made from the milk of cows that graze on fresh grass and hay. The texture of the cheese should be hard, almost gritty, and the flavor salty and slightly nutty. Parmigiano-Reggiano, which is named after the provinces where it is produced, is often aged for years before it is considered ready to eat.

1. Preheat the oven to 350°F.

2. Trim the cauliflower so that the white portion is intact and the leaves and stem are removed.

3. Place the cauliflower in a baking dish with about 1 cup of water, and cover the dish with foil.

4. Bake until the cauliflower is al dente, about 15 minutes.

5. While the cauliflower is baking, in a small bowl, stir together the Parmesan cheese, Mayonnaise, and Dijon mustard.

6. Transfer the cauliflower to a baking sheet, and coat the entire outside with the cheese mixture.

7. Place the cauliflower back in the oven, and bake until golden, about 15 minutes.

8. Serve.

PER SERVING: CALORIES: 141 / FAT: 12G / TOTAL CARBS: 6G
FIBER: 3G / NET CARBS: 3G / SUGAR: 2G / PROTEIN: 6G

Fat 76% / Carbs 12% / Protein 12%   Ratio: 2:1

1 large head cauliflower

½ cup grated Parmesan cheese

½ cup Mayonnaise (page 213)

1 tablespoon Dijon mustard

IN MENU FOR WEEK:

TRY INSTEAD: *The Dijon-and-cheese crust on this pretty side dish is delicious, but other ingredients are also wonderful. Tomato, crushed almonds, paprika, lemon juice, curry, and capers can all be used to flavor your cauliflower head.*

Fried Ham "Rice"

SERVES 4 / PREP TIME: 15 MINUTES / COOK TIME: 12 MINUTES

3 tablespoons toasted sesame oil

2 scallions, chopped

1 tablespoon grated fresh ginger

1 teaspoon minced garlic

½ cup ham, diced

3 large whole eggs, beaten

4 cups Cauliflower "Rice" (page 153)

¼ cup soy sauce

4 teaspoons toasted sesame seeds

1 tablespoon chopped fresh cilantro

Under 30 Minutes • One Pot *Fried rice can be found on every Chinese restaurant menu, and with good reason. The ingredient combination has a pleasing texture and a spectacularly balanced salty and spicy taste. Fresh ginger is essential for the subtle heat in the dish, so do not use ground ginger instead. Look for plump, unblemished ginger root in the produce section of the grocery store. Unpeeled ginger can last for up to 3 weeks in the refrigerator.*

1. In a large skillet over medium-high heat, heat the sesame oil.

2. Sauté the scallions, ginger, and garlic until softened, about 2 minutes.

3. Add the ham, and sauté for 1 minute.

4. Pour the beaten eggs into the skillet, and scramble them with the vegetables and ham until the eggs are cooked, about 3 minutes.

5. Stir in the Cauliflower "Rice" and soy sauce.

6. Sauté until all the ingredients are evenly mixed and heated through, about 5 minutes.

7. Topped with the sesame seeds and cilantro, and serve.

PER SERVING: CALORIES: 246 / FAT: 19G / TOTAL CARBS: 11G
FIBER: 5G / NET CARBS: 6G / SUGAR: 4G / PROTEIN: 12G

Fat 70% / Carbs 10% / Protein 20%   Ratio: 2:1

Stuffed Portobello Mushrooms

SERVES 4 / PREP TIME: 25 MINUTES / COOK TIME: 15 MINUTES

Make Ahead *Almond meal is practically identical to almond flour, except it has not been ground as long. The extra texture is wonderful in this mushroom stuffing. You can make your own almond meal by grinding up blanched almonds in a food processor until they are finely chopped. The timing is important because if you purée too long, you will end up with almond butter instead.*

1. Preheat the oven to 350°F.
2. Remove the stems from the mushroom caps, and use a spoon to scoop out the black gills to form a hollow. Set them aside on a small baking sheet.
3. In a medium skillet, heat the olive oil and sauté the garlic and kale until fragrant and the greens are tender, about 5 minutes.
4. Transfer the kale to a medium bowl, and stir in the cream cheese, basil, and pepper.
5. Mound the cheese mixture into the mushroom caps, and top each with 1 teaspoon of almond meal and 1 tablespoon of mozzarella cheese.
6. Bake the caps until the filling is heated through and the cheese is bubbly and golden, about 15 minutes, and serve.

PER SERVING: CALORIES: 300 / FAT: 25G / TOTAL CARBS: 9G
FIBER: 3G / NET CARBS: 6G / SUGAR: 0G / PROTEIN: 11G

Fat 75% / Carbs 11% / Protein 14%   Ratio: 2:1

4 portobello mushrooms

1 tablespoon extra-virgin olive oil

2 teaspoons minced garlic

1 cup shredded kale

1 cup cream cheese, softened

2 teaspoons chopped fresh basil

¼ teaspoon freshly ground black pepper

4 teaspoons almond meal, divided

¼ cup shredded mozzarella, divided

IN MENU FOR WEEKS:

A CLOSER LOOK: *Portobello mushrooms are often used as meat substitutes because of their dense texture and the variety of cooking applications that work well with this mushroom. They are high in protein, iron, potassium, copper, magnesium, and riboflavin. Portobello mushrooms can boost the immune system, decrease the risk of Alzheimer's disease, and support a healthy cardiovascular system.*

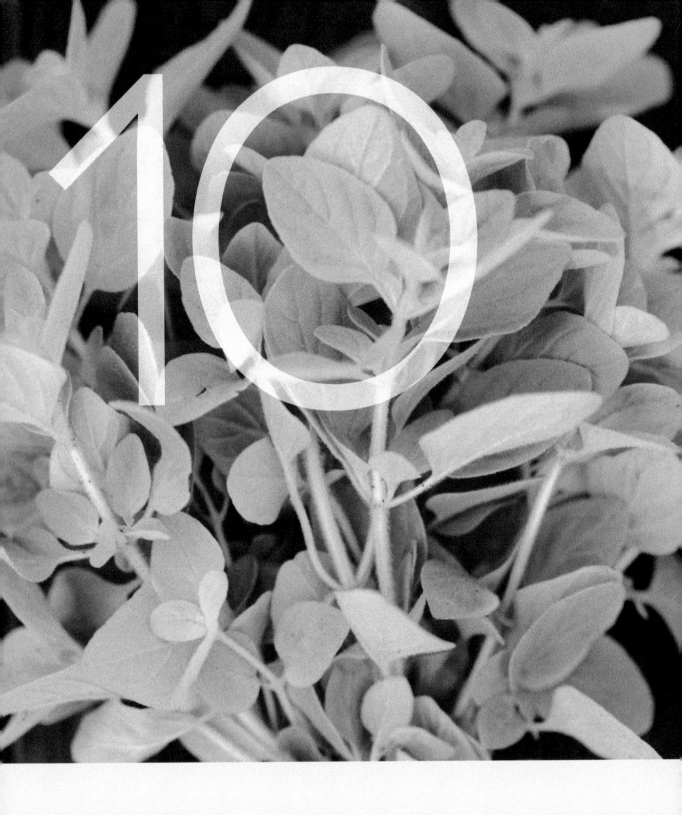

ENTRÉES

Barbecued Shrimp with Avocado Salsa

SERVES 4 / PREP TIME: 20 MINUTES, PLUS 2 HOURS TO MARINATE / COOK TIME: 8 MINUTES

FOR THE SHRIMP

1 pound (16–20 count) shrimp, peeled and deveined

2 tablespoons extra-virgin olive oil

1 tablespoon soy sauce

2 teaspoons minced garlic

1 teaspoon chili powder

FOR THE SALSA

1 avocado, peeled, pitted, and diced

6 sun-dried tomatoes (packed in oil), chopped

Juice and zest of 1 lime

1 scallion, chopped

1 tablespoon chopped fresh cilantro

1 teaspoon minced garlic

¼ cup goat cheese crumbles

IN MENU FOR WEEK:

A CLOSER LOOK: *Cilantro is high in antioxidants, potassium, and vitamins A, C, and K. This pretty, dark green herb can help reduce cholesterol levels, support a healthy cardiovascular system, and reduce the risk of Alzheimer's disease.*

Sun-dried tomatoes are available completely dried or packed in oil. The dried product usually has to be reconstituted with water before it can be used, and the oil-packed tomatoes add fat to this dish along with rich flavor. Sun-dried tomatoes contain as much lycopene as fresh tomatoes, which can help prevent prostate cancer and deadly pancreatic cancer. You can make your own "sun-dried" tomatoes in a 200°F oven if you toss tomato wedges with olive oil, spread them on a tray, and bake them until almost dried out.

TO MAKE THE SHRIMP

1. In a large bowl, toss together the shrimp, olive oil, soy sauce, garlic, and chili powder.

2. Refrigerate for 2 hours.

3. Take the shrimp out, and evenly divide them among 4 wooden skewers that have been soaked in water for 30 minutes.

4. Preheat the barbeque or a grill pan to medium heat.

5. Grill the shrimp, turning once, until they are opaque and cooked through, about 4 minutes per side.

TO MAKE THE SALSA

1. While the shrimp are cooking, in a medium bowl, mix together the avocado, sun-dried tomato, lime juice, lime zest, scallion, cilantro, and garlic.

2. Slide the cooked shrimp off the skewers, top with the salsa and crumbled goat cheese, and serve.

PER SERVING: CALORIES: 376 / FAT: 28G / TOTAL CARBS: 8G
FIBER: 4G / NET CARBS: 4G / SUGAR: 0G / PROTEIN: 26G

Fat 68% / Carbs 5% / Protein 27%   Ratio: 2:1

Sea Scallops with Bacon Cream Sauce

SERVES 4 / PREP TIME: 15 MINUTES / COOK TIME: 20 MINUTES

Scallops have a mild, sweet taste with absolutely no fishy overtones, so even those who do not enjoy seafood can dig into this dish with abandon. Scallops are very high in vitamin B_{12}, iodine, potassium, protein, and selenium.

1. In a saucepan over medium-high heat, cook the bacon, stirring, until it is crispy, about 5 minutes. Using a slotted spoon, remove the cooked bacon to a plate.

2. Sauté the onions and garlic in the bacon fat until softened, about 3 minutes.

3. Add the white wine, and deglaze the saucepan, stirring to scrape up the browned bits from the bottom.

4. Whisk in the heavy cream and reserved bacon, and bring the mixture to a simmer.

5. Simmer until the sauce thickens, about 5 minutes.

6. Remove the sauce from the heat, and stir in the thyme. Set aside.

7. In a large nonstick skillet over medium-high heat, heat the olive oil. Season the scallops with salt and pepper.

8. Cook the scallops undisturbed until the bottoms are browned and crisped, about 3 minutes.

9. Using tongs, carefully turn the scallops, and sear the other side until they are also browned and crisped, 3 minutes longer.

10. Transfer the seared scallops to a plate, and serve with the sauce.

6 bacon slices, chopped

½ small onion, chopped fine

1 teaspoon minced garlic

¼ cup dry white wine

1 cup heavy (whipping) cream

1 teaspoon chopped fresh thyme

1 tablespoon extra-virgin olive oil

1 pound sea scallops, washed, cleaned, and dried thoroughly

Sea salt

Freshly ground black pepper

IN MENU FOR WEEK:

PER SERVING: CALORIES: 410 / FAT: 32G / TOTAL CARBS: 5G
FIBER: 0G / NET CARBS: 5G / SUGAR: 2G / PROTEIN: 25G

Fat 70% / Carbs 6% / Protein 24%   Ratio: 2:1

Spicy Crab Cakes

SERVES 4 / PREP TIME: 20 MINUTES, PLUS 1 HOUR TO CHILL / COOK TIME: 20 MINUTES

1 pound crab

½ cup almond flour, plus additional for dusting

½ red bell pepper, minced

¼ cup Mayonnaise (page 213)

3 tablespoons minced red onion

1 teaspoon Dijon mustard

1 teaspoon Worcestershire sauce

1 teaspoon chopped fresh dill

Splash Tabasco sauce

3 tablespoons extra-virgin olive oil

IN MENU FOR WEEK:

 3

A CLOSER LOOK: *Dill is a flamboyant herb with plumy green fronds and an abundance of tiny yellow flowers. The bunches available in the supermarket are enormous, so it is lucky dill is so healthy and works so well in many recipes. Eating dill can protect you from free radicals and carcinogens.*

Make Ahead *Crab is low in calories and high in protein, omega-3 fatty acids, chromium, and selenium. This sweet crustacean can help support cardiovascular health, boost the immune system, lower the risk of cancer, and reduce inflammation in the body. You can use canned crab if fresh or frozen is not available, but avoid imitation crab made with pollack and food coloring.*

1. In a large bowl, stir together the crab, almond flour, red pepper, Mayonnaise, red onion, Dijon mustard, Worcestershire sauce, dill, and Tabasco sauce until the mixture holds together when pressed.

2. Form the crab mixture into 12 patties, and refrigerate them on a plate, covered, for 1 hour. Dust with additional almond flour.

3. In a large skillet over medium-high heat, heat the olive oil.

4. Cook the crab cakes in batches, until golden brown and heated through, about 10 minutes per side.

5. Serve.

———————

PER SERVING: CALORIES: 349 / FAT: 29G / TOTAL CARBS: 6G
FIBER: 2G / NET CARBS: 4G / SUGAR: 2G / PROTEIN: 16G

Fat 75% / Carbs 6% / Protein 19%   Ratio: 2:1

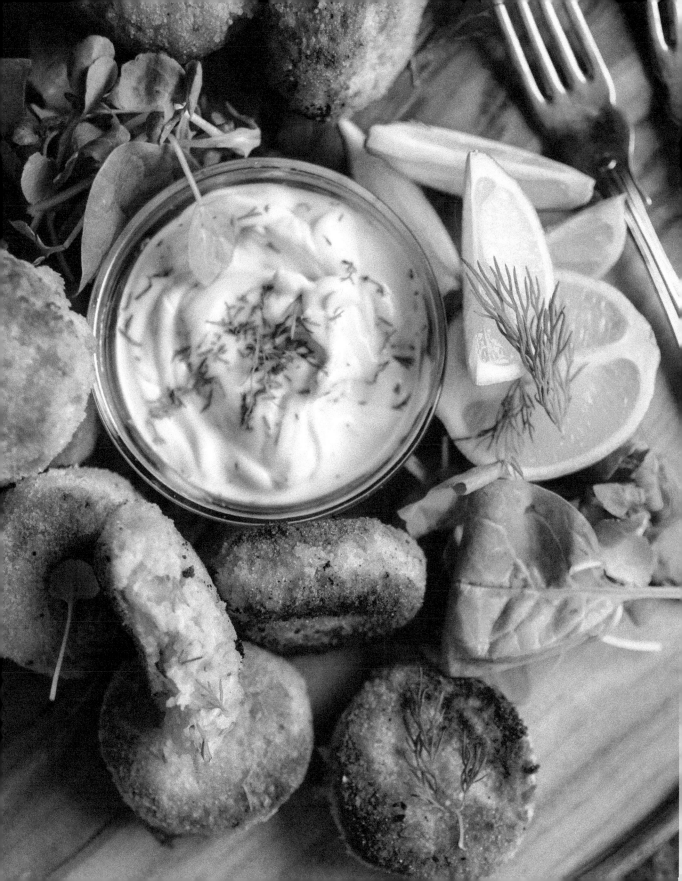

Brown Butter–Lime Tilapia

SERVES 4 / PREP TIME: 10 MINUTES / COOK TIME: 15 MINUTES

½ cup unsalted butter

¼ cup chopped fresh dill

Juice of 1 lime

4 (4-ounce) tilapia fillets

Sea salt

Freshly ground
black pepper

4 teaspoons coconut oil

IN MENU FOR WEEK:

4

Under 30 Minutes *Tilapia is readily available in supermarkets because it is a popular choice for those who farm fish. Tilapia has a mild taste and firm white flesh, so most cooking methods and other ingredients work well. Tilapia is very high in protein and very low in carbohydrates and fat. So, a sauce made almost entirely with butter is a perfect accompaniment to add the fat required in the keto lifestyle.*

1. In a small saucepan over medium-high heat, heat the butter until it starts to foam up and fizz. Swirl the saucepan until tiny brown specks form and the butter smells nutty, about 1 minute.

2. Remove from the heat, and set aside.

3. In a blender, purée the dill and lime juice until a paste forms.

4. Slowly pour the brown butter into the blender while it is running until an emulsified sauce forms and all the butter is used.

5. Rinse the tilapia fillets, and pat them dry with paper towels.

6. Season the fish lightly with salt and pepper on both sides.

7. In a large skillet over medium-high heat, heat the coconut oil.

8. Brown the fish on both sides, turning once, for about 10 minutes total.

9. Serve the fish with the brown butter sauce immediately.

PER SERVING: CALORIES: 347 / FAT: 28G / TOTAL CARBS: 3G
FIBER: 1G / NET CARBS: 2G / SUGAR: 0G / PROTEIN: 22G

Fat 73% / Carbs 2% / Protein 25%   Ratio: 2:1

Sole Meunière

SERVES 4 / PREP TIME: 15 MINUTES / COOK TIME: 10 MINUTES

Under 30 Minutes • One Pot *The crowning touch to the famous meunière sauce is a generous amount of fresh parsley. Most often seen lying limply on the side of plates as a garnish, this perky herb is packed with nutrients such as vitamins C and K, chlorophyll, beta-carotene, magnesium, and iron. Parsley can help purify the blood, support eye health, and reduce the risk of cancer, stroke, and diabetes. Parsley can be very gritty, so make sure you soak the sprigs in a bowlful of water to remove all the dirt before drying and chopping it.*

1. Pat the fish almost dry with paper towels, and season both sides with salt and pepper.

2. On a large plate, dredge the sole in the almond flour.

3. In a large skillet over medium-high heat, heat 6 table-spoons of butter.

4. Swirl the skillet until the butter starts to foam and brown flecks appear, about 1 minute.

5. Reduce the heat to medium-low, and add the fish fillets to the skillet.

6. Fry the fish until browned on both sides, turning once, about 6 minutes in total.

7. Remove the fish from the skillet, and transfer them to plates.

8. Stir in the remaining butter, lemon juice, lemon zest, parsley, and thyme.

9. Whisk over the heat for 2 minutes, and then serve the fish with the buttery sauce.

4 (4-ounce) sole fillets

Sea salt

Freshly ground black pepper

½ cup almond flour

½ cup butter, divided

Juice and zest of 3 lemons

½ cup chopped fresh parsley

1 teaspoon fresh chopped thyme

IN MENU FOR WEEKS:

A CLOSER LOOK: *This classic dish can be traced to Normandy, but it found fame as Julia Child's first meal in France and the inspiration for her culinary journey. The perfection of the dish is found in a few quality ingredients prepared beautifully.*

PER SERVING: CALORIES: 435 / FAT: 33G / TOTAL CARBS: 4G
FIBER: 2G / NET CARBS: 2G / SUGAR: 1G / PROTEIN: 28G

Fat 70% / Carbs 5% / Protein 25%   Ratio: 2:1

Golden Fried Fish

SERVES 4 / PREP TIME: 15 MINUTES / COOK TIME: 12 MINUTES

1 pound boneless haddock fillets, cut into 4 equal pieces

¼ cup almond flour, divided

1 egg

1 tablespoon water

½ cup Parmesan cheese

¼ cup flaxseed meal

¼ teaspoon freshly ground black pepper

Pinch ground cayenne pepper

½ cup extra-virgin olive oil

Lemon wedges, for garnish

IN MENU FOR WEEK:

Under 30 Minutes *Haddock is a firm white-flesh fish that flakes off in large, moist chunks when cooked. You will want to see almost translucent, firm flesh rather than fish that looks opaque. An opaque fish means it is not as fresh. The raw haddock should smell fresh rather than fishy as well.*

1. Pat the fish dry with paper towels, and set aside.

2. Put 2 tablespoons of almond flour in a small bowl, and set it next to the fish.

3. In another small bowl, stir together the eggs and water, and set the mixture next to the almond flour.

4. In a medium bowl, stir together the remaining 2 tablespoons of almond flour with the Parmesan cheese, flaxseed meal, black pepper, and cayenne pepper. Set the bowl next to the egg mixture.

5. Dredge the fish pieces in the almond flour, the egg mixture, and the flour mixture, in that order, until all 4 pieces are coated.

6. In a large skillet over medium-high heat, heat the olive oil.

7. When the oil is hot, fry the fish, turning once, until both sides are golden and crispy and the fish is cooked through, about 6 minutes per side, depending on the thickness of the fish.

8. Transfer the fish to a paper towel-lined plate, and use paper towels to blot off the excess oil.

9. Serve with the lemon wedges.

PER SERVING: CALORIES: 349 / FAT: 25G / TOTAL CARBS: 4G
FIBER: 3G / NET CARBS: 1G / SUGAR: 1G / PROTEIN: 27G

Fat 65% / Carbs 4% / Protein 31%   Ratio: 1:1

Baked Halibut with Herb Sauce

SERVES 4 / PREP TIME: 15 MINUTES / COOK TIME: 18 MINUTES

For a dish that takes about 30 minutes from start to finish, the presentation is absolutely spectacular. People will think you spent hours slaving over a hot stove. Halibut can be difficult to get because it has been overfished in the Atlantic Ocean, so the best source is Pacific halibut, which is usually sustainably fished and uncontaminated. Always inquire about the origins of the fish you purchase, and look for halibut from Canadian, Alaskan, and California fisheries.

1. Preheat the oven to 400°F.

2. Line a baking sheet with parchment paper, and set aside.

3. Pat the fish dry with paper towels, and lightly oil all the pieces with the olive oil.

4. Season both sides of the fish with salt and pepper.

5. Place the fillets on the baking sheet, and bake until cooked through, about 15 to 18 minutes.

6. While the fish is cooking, in a small bowl, stir together the yogurt, Mayonnaise, sour cream, lemon juice, lemon zest, dill, basil, and chives.

7. Serve the fish with a generous dollop of sauce.

PER SERVING: CALORIES: 374 / FAT: 25G / TOTAL CARBS: 2G
FIBER: 0G / NET CARBS: 2G / SUGAR: 1G / PROTEIN: 33G

Fat 60% / Carbs 5% / Protein 35%   Ratio: 2:1

4 (5-ounce) halibut fillets

1 tablespoon extra-virgin olive oil

Sea salt

Freshly ground black pepper

½ cup plain Greek yogurt

¼ cup Mayonnaise (page 213)

2 tablespoons sour cream

Juice and zest of 1 lemon

1 tablespoon chopped fresh dill

1 teaspoon chopped fresh basil

1 teaspoon chopped fresh chives

IN MENU FOR WEEK:

4

KITCHEN HACK: *The creamy, fragrant sauce found in this dish will keep in the fridge for up to 2 weeks in a sealed container. You do not have to buy bunches of herbs that will wilt unused in your refrigerator for this sauce because any combination will be lovely. Use whatever herbs you have on hand in your kitchen or garden.*

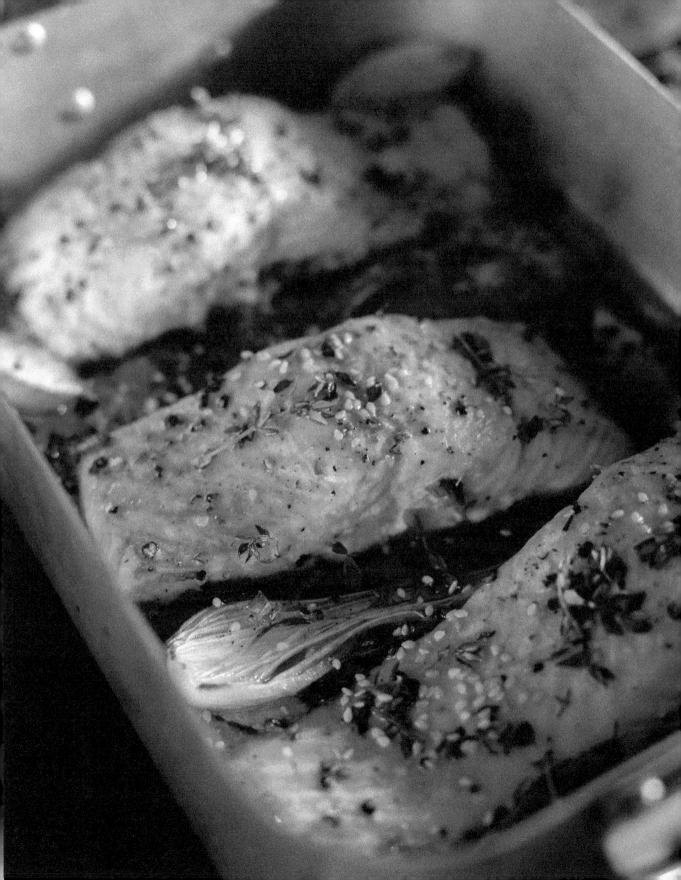

Sesame Salmon

SERVES 4 / PREP TIME: 15 MINUTES / COOK TIME: 15 MINUTES

Under 30 Minutes *The salmon in most grocery stores is farmed unless specified as wild caught. Wild-caught salmon is a better option because it contains more omega-3 fatty acids and is organic. It is more expensive than farmed, and the price tag on wild-hooked salmon can be shocking. The flesh of salmon can vary extensively in color, depending on whether it is farmed or wild. Farmed salmon has a pale pink hue unless deliberately dyed, and wild salmon is a gorgeous rich, deep red. Salmon is very high in heart-friendly fats, protein, and vitamin D. This fish can help lower blood pressure, decrease inflammation in the joints, and improve brain and nerve health.*

Olive oil, for greasing

2 tablespoons soy sauce

2 tablespoons rice vinegar

4 teaspoons sesame oil

4 (5-ounce) boneless salmon fillets

Sea salt

Freshly ground black pepper

¼ cup sesame seeds

2 teaspoons chopped fresh thyme

1. Preheat the oven to 425°F.

2. Lightly oil a 9-by-13-inch baking dish with olive oil, and set aside.

3. In a small bowl, whisk together the soy sauce, rice vinegar, and sesame oil.

4. Pat the salmon dry with paper towels, and lightly season both sides of the fillets with salt and pepper.

5. Place the salmon in the baking dish.

6. Pour the soy mixture over the salmon, and bake the fish in the oven until it is just cooked through, about 13 to 15 minutes.

7. Top the salmon with sesame seeds and chopped thyme, and serve.

PER SERVING: CALORIES: 303 / FAT: 19G / TOTAL CARBS: 3G
FIBER: 1G / NET CARBS: 2G / SUGAR: 0G / PROTEIN: 30G

Fat 56% / Carbs 3% / Protein 41%   Ratio: 1:2

Caprese Balsamic Chicken

SERVES 4 / PREP TIME: 10 MINUTES / COOK TIME: 25 MINUTES

3 tablespoons
balsamic vinegar

1 tablespoon butter

2 (6-ounce) boneless,
skinless chicken breasts,
halved lengthwise

Sea salt

Freshly ground
black pepper

1 tablespoon extra-virgin
olive oil

¼ cup Herb Pesto
(page 219), divided

1 tomato, cut into 4 slices

1 cup shredded
mozzarella cheese

IN MENU FOR WEEKS:

A CLOSER LOOK: *There is
more to mozzarella than the
pale, stringy topping found
on almost every pizza in
North America. Traditional
mozzarella is a curd cheese
made from water buffalo
milk and eaten fresh only a
few hours after it is made.
The whey is removed, and
the strings of curd are
strung and cut, creating the
distinctive texture.*

*Balsamic vinegar is unique and not like other vinegars at all. It
is a reduction created by boiling down grape pressings and aged
under strict parameters, often for between 12 and 100 years.
Other vinegars are created from fermented wine. The balsamic
vinegar you purchase in the grocery store is probably not true
balsamic vinegar, unless you spend several hundred dollars
for it. Many products labeled as balsamic are actually other
types of vinegars with coloring and flavor added, but even the
less-than-authentic products still taste lovely when you use them
in your recipes.*

1. Preheat the oven to 400°F.

2. In a small saucepan over medium heat, bring the
   balsamic vinegar and butter to a boil; then reduce
   the heat to low and simmer until thickened, about
   5 minutes. Set aside.

3. Season the chicken breasts with salt and pepper.

4. In a medium skillet over medium heat, heat the olive oil.

5. Cook the chicken, turning once, until just cooked
   through, about 10 minutes total.

6. Place the cooked chicken in a 9-by-13-baking dish.

7. Spread 1 tablespoon of pesto over each piece of chicken,
   top each with tomato slices, and evenly divide the
   cheese between the pieces.

8. Bake in the oven until the cheese is melted and golden,
   about 5 minutes.

9. Serve with a drizzle of the reduced balsamic vinegar.

PER SERVING: CALORIES: 375 / FAT: 25G / TOTAL CARBS: 3G
FIBER: 0G / NET CARBS: 3G / SUGAR: 1G / PROTEIN: 35G

Fat 60% / Carbs 3% / Protein 37%   Ratio: 1:1

Coconut Chicken

SERVES 4 / PREP TIME: 15 MINUTES, PLUS 2 HOURS TO MARINATE / COOK TIME: 20 MINUTES

Curried chicken is the choice of people all over the world for intimate dinners for two, rousing get-togethers with friends, and those nights when you just want to curl up on the couch alone to watch a beloved movie. One of the spices that contribute to the glorious flavor of the dish is cumin. Cumin has a strong, nutty, peppery flavor and it is very high in iron, manganese, calcium, and magnesium.

1. Cut each chicken breast on an angle into 4 pieces, and put the chicken into a sealable freezer bag.

2. In a medium bowl, whisk together the coconut milk, soy sauce, stevia, curry, cumin, coriander, and cayenne.

3. Pour one-quarter of the sauce into the bag with the chicken. Seal the bag, pressing out the air, and refrigerate the chicken to marinate for 2 hours.

4. Pour the remaining sauce into a small saucepan over medium heat.

5. Bring the sauce to a boil, reduce the heat to low, and simmer until the sauce is thick, about 10 minutes.

6. Remove the sauce from the heat, and set aside.

7. In a large skillet over medium-high heat, heat the coconut oil.

8. Remove the chicken from the marinade, and sauté it, turning once, until it is cooked through and golden, about 5 minutes per side.

9. Top with the cilantro and lime wedges, and serve with the sauce.

2 (8-ounce) boneless, skinless chicken breasts

1 cup coconut milk

2 tablespoons soy sauce

1 (7g) stevia packet

2 teaspoons curry powder

1 teaspoon ground cumin

1 teaspoon ground coriander

Pinch ground cayenne pepper

3 tablespoons coconut oil

¼ cup chopped fresh cilantro

1 lime, cut into wedges

IN MENU FOR WEEK:

2

PER SERVING: CALORIES: 453 / FAT: 33G / TOTAL CARBS: 5G
FIBER: 2G / NET CARBS: 3G / SUGAR: 2G / PROTEIN: 35G

Fat 66% / Carbs 4% / Protein 30%   Ratio: 1:1

Chicken Milanese

SERVES 4 / PREP TIME: 30 MINUTES / COOK TIME: 40 MINUTES

FOR THE SAUCE

2 tablespoons butter

½ scallion, chopped

¼ cup dry white wine

½ cup chicken stock

½ cup heavy (whipping) cream

1 teaspoon thyme

1 teaspoon freshly squeezed lemon juice

FOR THE CHICKEN

2 (8-ounce) chicken breasts, halved lengthwise

¾ cup almond flour

¼ cup Parmesan cheese

1 large egg

1 tablespoon water

¼ cup extra-virgin olive oil

¼ cup chopped fresh parsley

IN MENU FOR WEEKS:

Breading chicken, or any food, can be an extremely messy activity, and you might end up with completely breaded fingers at the end of the process. A professional chef trick for avoiding this issue is to have a wet hand and a dry hand. Only use the left (or right) hand to dip the chicken in the egg mixture and the other hand for the dry ingredients. Make sure you drop the poultry into each dish without touching the contents, and most of the breading ingredients will end up on the chicken where it belongs.

TO MAKE THE SAUCE

1. In a medium saucepan over medium-high heat, melt the butter.

2. Sauté the scallion until it is bright green, about 2 minutes.

3. Add the wine, chicken stock, and cream.

4. Bring the sauce to a boil, reduce the heat to low, and simmer until the sauce reduces to about 1 cup, about 20 minutes.

5. Remove the sauce from the heat, and stir in the thyme and lemon juice. Set aside.

TO MAKE THE CHICKEN

1. Use a mallet to pound the chicken pieces out thin without ripping through. Pat the pieces dry with paper towels.

2. In a large bowl, stir the almond flour and Parmesan cheese together.

3. In another small bowl, stir the egg and water together.

4. Dip the chicken pieces in the egg mixture, and then dredge them in the almond-cheese mixture to coat.

5. In a large skillet over medium heat, heat the olive oil.

6. In a large skillet, cook the breaded chicken pieces until the bottom is golden brown, about 3 minutes.

7. Turn the cutlets over, and cook until the chicken is cooked through and the second side is golden brown, about 4 minutes.

8. Top the cutlets with the parsley, and serve with the sauce.

PER SERVING: CALORIES: 542 / FAT: 41G / TOTAL CARBS: 6G
FIBER: 3G / NET CARBS: 3G / SUGAR: 1G / PROTEIN: 32G

Fat 70% / Carbs 5% / Protein 25%　Ratio: 2:1

Herb-Infused Chicken

SERVES 4 / PREP TIME: 15 MINUTES / COOK TIME: 35 MINUTES

3 tablespoons extra-virgin olive oil, divided

4 (7-ounce) chicken thighs, bone in

½ cup green olives

Juice of 2 lemons

1 teaspoon lemon zest

1 teaspoon minced garlic

1 teaspoon chopped fresh tarragon

1 teaspoon chopped fresh thyme

1 teaspoon chopped fresh rosemary

IN MENU FOR WEEK:

3

A CLOSER LOOK: *Olive oil is made by pressing whole olives, and this oil has been produced for thousands of years as a beauty aid as well as for medicinal and culinary uses. Consuming olive oil every day can reduce many of the factors that contribute to heart disease, boost the immune system, and help prevent cancer.*

One Pot *Tarragon is a very popular herb in Mediterranean cuisine. This delicate aromatic herb has a distinct anise or licorice flavor and is a good source of antioxidants and phytonutrients. Tarragon contains iron, calcium, potassium, and vitamin A. It was used as a folk medicine for stimulating appetite, but it can also support the cardiovascular system and promote healthy eyes.*

1. Preheat the oven to 450°F.

2. In a large ovenproof skillet over medium heat, heat 1 tablespoon of olive oil.

3. Sear the chicken thighs for 4 minutes per side.

4. Remove the skillet from the heat, and use a fork to prick the chicken thighs all over.

5. In a small bowl, stir the remaining 2 tablespoons of olive oil together with the green olives, lemon juice, lemon zest, garlic, tarragon, thyme, and rosemary.

6. Add the olive oil mixture to the chicken, cover the skillet, and place it in the oven.

7. Braise the chicken thighs until they are cooked through and tender, about 25 minutes, and serve.

PER SERVING: CALORIES: 435 / FAT: 36G / TOTAL CARBS: 2G
FIBER: 1G / NET CARBS: 1G / SUGAR: 0G / PROTEIN: 26G

Fat 74% / Carbs 2% / Protein 24%   Ratio: 2:1

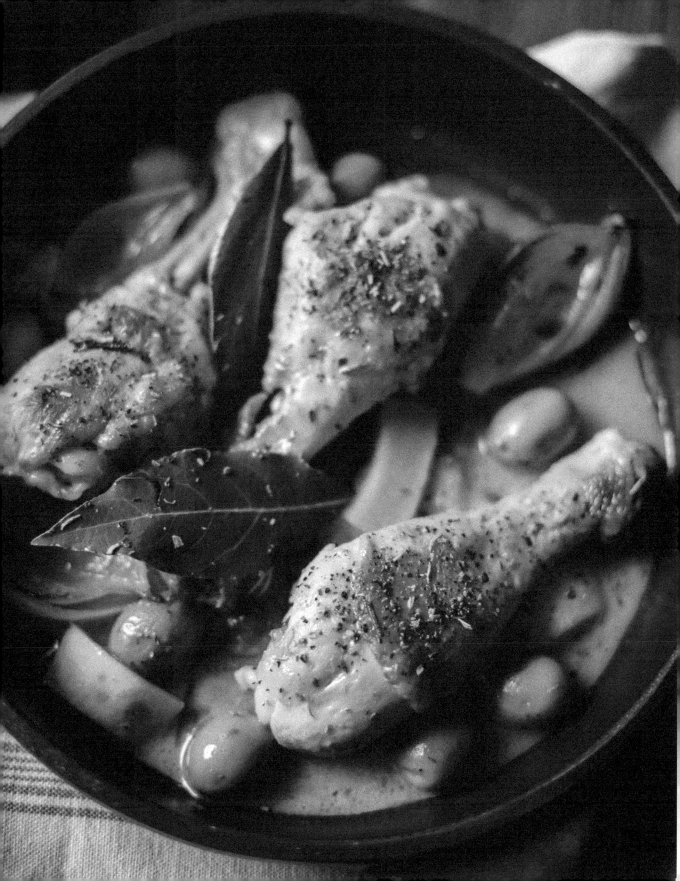

Rich Sausage Casserole

SERVES 4 / PREP TIME: 15 MINUTES / COOK TIME: 40 MINUTES

Butter, for greasing

½ pound pork sausage meat

2 cups cooked spaghetti squash

1 tomato, chopped

1 jalapeño pepper, minced

4 large eggs, beaten

½ cup shredded aged Cheddar cheese

¼ cup chopped cilantro

IN MENU FOR WEEK:

1

TRY INSTEAD: *The taste in this casserole can change depending on the sausage you use in the dish. Sausage can be made from any meat including turkey, beef, pork, venison, chicken, and wild game. Try different types of sausage to create unique casseroles for any occasion.*

Make Ahead *Part of the delicious appeal of this bubbly casserole is the rich Cheddar cheese. Cheddar comes in a dizzying variety of ages, colors, and additives because unlike other cheeses, the term Cheddar is not regulated, so it can be applied to many cheeses. Cheddar is naturally a pale yellow or white, so avoid any colored bright orange with dyes. The flavor of Cheddar gets sharper as it ages, so look for one that is at least 2 years old for this recipe.*

1. Preheat the oven to 350°F.

2. Lightly grease an 8-cup casserole dish with butter, and set aside.

3. In a large skillet over medium heat, sauté the sausage meat until cooked through.

4. Add the squash, tomato, and jalapeño to the skillet, and stir.

5. Sauté the mixture until most of the liquid has evaporated, about 10 minutes.

6. Remove the skillet from the heat, and stir in the eggs.

7. Transfer the mixture to the casserole dish, and sprinkle with the cheese.

8. Bake until the casserole is set and the top is golden and bubbly, about 30 minutes.

9. Top with the cilantro, and serve.

PER SERVING: CALORIES: 307 / FAT: 24G / TOTAL CARBS: 5G
FIBER: 0G / NET CARBS: 4G / SUGAR: 1G / PROTEIN: 18G

Fat 70% / Carbs 7% / Protein 23%   Ratio: 2:1

Ham-Stuffed Pork Chops

SERVES 4 / PREP TIME: 15 MINUTES / COOK TIME: 40 MINUTES

You can use peameal bacon or other types of cheese in the stuffing, but don't overstuff or it will be impossible to bread the pork chop completely. You want to have a completely enclosed chop so that the melted cheese does not ooze out until you cut it open on your plate.

1. Preheat the oven to 350°F. Cut the pork chops horizontally throughout the middle without cutting right through, to create a pocket.

2. Stuff each pork chop with a slice of Swiss cheese and a slice of ham.

3. Seal the edges of the meat with toothpicks.

4. In a large bowl, dredge the pork chops in the almond flour.

5. Add the Parmesan cheese to the almond flour left in the bowl, and stir to combine.

6. In another large bowl, stir together the egg and water, and dip the pork chops in the egg mixture, shaking off the excess.

7. Dredge the meat in the almond flour-cheese mixture to completely coat.

8. In a large skillet over medium heat, heat the olive oil.

9. Brown the pork chops on both sides until golden brown, about 4 minutes per side.

10. Place the pork chops in a baking dish, and bake until cooked through, about 30 to 35 minutes.

11. Serve.

4 (4-ounce) pork chops, center cut, about 1 inch thick

4 slices Swiss cheese

4 slices black forest ham

¾ cup almond flour

½ cup Parmesan cheese

1 large egg

1 tablespoon water

2 tablespoons extra-virgin olive oil

IN MENU FOR WEEKS:

PER SERVING: CALORIES: 491 / FAT: 33G / TOTAL CARBS: 6G
FIBER: 3G / NET CARBS: 3G / SUGAR: 1G / PROTEIN: 38G

Fat 63% / Carbs 5% / Protein 32%   Ratio: 1:1

Swedish Meatballs

SERVES 6 / PREP TIME: 15 MINUTES / COOK TIME: 25 MINUTES

FOR THE MEATBALLS

2 tablespoons extra-virgin olive oil, divided

1 onion, diced

½ teaspoon minced garlic

¾ pound ground beef

¾ pound ground pork

2 tablespoons coconut flour

1 egg

¼ teaspoon ground allspice

¼ teaspoon ground nutmeg

FOR THE SAUCE

¼ cup unsalted butter

3 tablespoons arrowroot

4 cups beef broth

1 cup sour cream

Sea salt

Freshly ground black pepper

2 tablespoons chopped fresh parsley leaves

IN MENU FOR WEEK:

2

Swedish meatballs, or köttbullar, are probably the most famous dish from this region of the world, and originally the meatball component was created to use up leftovers. This is why recipes often use different meats such as beef, lamb, and pork, as well as an assortment of fillers. This recipe uses both beef and pork to create a more complex flavor, but you can simply choose one.

TO MAKE THE MEATBALLS

1. In a large skillet over medium heat, heat 1 tablespoon of olive oil.

2. Sauté the onion and garlic until softened, about 3 minutes.

3. Transfer the vegetables to a large bowl.

4. Add the ground beef, ground pork, coconut flour, egg, allspice, and nutmeg to the bowl, and mix to combine.

5. Roll the mixture into 1-inch balls; you should get about 24 in total.

6. Wipe the skillet out with a paper towel, and add the remaining 1 tablespoon of olive oil.

7. Place the skillet over medium heat, and brown the meatballs in batches until they are fully browned, about 5 minutes per batch.

8. Set the browned meatballs aside on a plate.

TO MAKE THE SAUCE

1. In a large skillet, melt the butter. Whisk in the arrowroot to form a paste.

2. Whisk in the beef broth, and cook until the sauce is thickened, about 2 minutes.

3. Whisk in the sour cream, and season the sauce with salt and pepper.

4. Add the meatballs back to the sauce, and cook until they are heated completely through, about 10 minutes.

5. Top with the parsley, and serve.

PER SERVING: CALORIES: 435 / FAT: 29G / TOTAL CARBS: 6G
FIBER: 2G / NET CARBS: 4G / SUGAR: 2G / PROTEIN: 38G

Fat 60% / Carbs 5% / Protein 35%   Ratio: 1:2

Casserole au Gratin

SERVES 4 / PREP TIME: 25 MINUTES / COOK TIME: 30 MINUTES

4 tablespoons butter, melted, plus more for greasing

5 cups cauliflower, cut into small florets

2 cups diced lean ham

4 ounces cream cheese, softened

½ cup Greek yogurt

1 jalapeño pepper, diced

1 scallion, chopped

1 cup almond flour

1 teaspoon chopped fresh parsley

IN MENU FOR WEEKS:

Make Ahead *Cream cheese is the magic ingredient that creates an addictive, decadent, smooth sauce. Cream cheese is unripened cheese made from cow's milk, and USDA law stipulates that regular cream cheese is 33 percent fat. You will only be using about ½ cup of cheese, so use the rest in other recipes because the cheese will only keep about a week after opened. Cream cheese is lovely in omelets, baking, pâté, meatballs, sauces, and ice cream.*

1. Preheat the oven to 350°F.

2. Lightly butter an 8-cup casserole dish.

3. Place a large saucepan filled with water over high heat, and bring the water to a boil.

4. Blanch the cauliflower until it is tender-crisp, about 4 minutes.

5. Drain the cauliflower, and transfer it to a large bowl.

6. Add the ham to the bowl and toss to combine.

7. In a small bowl, whisk together the cream cheese, yogurt, jalapeño, and scallion until well mixed.

8. Stir the cream cheese mixture into the cauliflower mixture, mixing to coat the vegetables and ham.

9. Spoon the mixture into the casserole dish.

10. In a small bowl, stir together the almond flour, butter, and parsley until the mixture looks like coarse crumbs.

11. Sprinkle the topping over the casserole evenly.

12. Bake until the topping is lightly browned and all the mixture is bubbly, about 20 minutes.

13. Serve.

PER SERVING: CALORIES: 501 / FAT: 38G / TOTAL CARBS: 14G
FIBER: 7G / NET CARBS: 7G / SUGAR: 5G / PROTEIN: 20G

Fat 70% / Carbs 12% / Protein 18%   Ratio: 2:1

Pan-Grilled Lamb Chops with Herb Pesto

SERVES 4 / PREP TIME: 10 MINUTES / COOK TIME: 20 MINUTES

Under 30 Minutes • One Pot *Take a little extra time to source exceptional lamb, under 1 year old, to get the most flavor and health benefits. Look for firm, pink flesh with white fat marbling, not yellow. Organic, grass-fed meat contains more omega-3 fatty acids because these levels are dependent on what the animal eats. Even "regular" lamb is very high in vitamin B$_{12}$, protein, selenium, and vitamin B$_3$. Eating lamb can reduce your risk of heart disease and can help regulate blood sugar.*

1. Season the lamb chops with salt and pepper.

2. Let the lamb chops sit, covered, until they reach room temperature.

3. In a large skillet over medium-high heat, heat the olive oil.

4. Sear the chops in the skillet for about 5 minutes on each side for medium-rare.

5. Let the lamb chops rest for 10 minutes before serving them with 1 tablespoon of Herb Pesto for each chop.

4 (4-ounce) lamb chops

Sea salt

Freshly ground black pepper

2 tablespoons extra-virgin olive oil

¼ cup Herb Pesto (page 219), divided

IN MENU FOR WEEK:

 3

PER SERVING: CALORIES: 413 / FAT: 32G / TOTAL CARBS: 2G
FIBER: 2G / NET CARBS: 0G / SUGAR: 0G / PROTEIN: 32G

Fat 70% / Carbs 0% / Protein 30%   Ratio: 1:1

Bacon-Wrapped Beef Tenderloin

SERVES 4 / PREP TIME: 10 MINUTES / COOK TIME: 20 MINUTES

4 (4-ounce)
beef tenderloin steaks

Sea salt

Freshly ground
black pepper

12 bacon slices

2 tablespoons extra-virgin
olive oil

IN MENU FOR WEEK:

TRY INSTEAD: *Many people*
are obsessed with salty,
rich bacon, so wrapping
it around a steak is not
unusual. However, bacon
has variations in flavor
and texture depending
on the curing process, so
experimentation can pro-
duce different results. Try
applewood-smoked bacon
to elevate this dish to a
culinary triumph.

Under 30 Minutes • One Pot *Beef tenderloin is one of the prime cuts you can purchase because it comes from a part of the cow right beneath the ribs and next to the backbone. This muscle does not move very much, so the meat is tender, fine-grained, and not as flavorful as less favorable cuts. Look for tenderloin that is butchered cleanly with all the silver skin removed smoothly.*

1. Preheat the oven to 450°F.

2. Pat the steaks dry with paper towels, and season them on all sides with salt and pepper.

3. Wrap each steak with 3 slices of bacon around the edges, overlapping the strips, and secure the bacon with toothpicks.

4. In a large skillet over medium-high heat, heat the olive oil.

5. Sear the steaks on each side for 4 minutes.

6. Place the steaks on a baking tray, and roast them in the oven for 5 to 6 minutes for medium doneness.

7. Remove the steaks from the oven, and let the meat rest for 10 minutes.

8. Remove the toothpicks, and serve.

PER SERVING: CALORIES: 396 / FAT: 25G / TOTAL CARBS: 0G
FIBER: 0G / NET CARBS: 0G / SUGAR: 0G / PROTEIN: 40G

Fat 60% / Carbs 0% / Protein 40%   Ratio: 1:2

Italian Meatballs

SERVES 4 / PREP TIME: 20 MINUTES / COOK TIME: 20 MINUTES

Make Ahead *The tiny pinch of allspice might not seem important, but you will miss the flavor in the finished meatballs if you leave it out. This spice comes from the unripe fruit of an evergreen tropical shrub. Allspice is a warm spice high in vitamin C, iron, calcium, magnesium, copper, manganese, iron, and magnesium. Allspice can reduce blood pressure, cut the risk of diabetes, and relieve symptoms associated with PMS and arthritis.*

1. Preheat the oven to 350°F.

2. Line a baking sheet with parchment, and set aside.

3. In a large bowl, mix together the ground beef, Parmesan, almond flour, egg, onion, garlic, basil, oregano, and allspice until well blended.

4. Roll the beef mixture into 1½-inch balls.

5. In a large skillet over medium-high heat, heat the oil.

6. Brown the meatballs in the skillet all over, for about 10 minutes, and transfer them to the baking sheet.

7. Bake the meatballs until just cooked through, about 10 minutes.

8. Serve plain or with your favorite sauce.

PER SERVING: CALORIES: 480 / FAT: 38G / TOTAL CARBS: 6G
FIBER: 2G / NET CARBS: 4G / SUGAR: 1G / PROTEIN: 34G

Fat 71% / Carbs 3% / Protein 27%   Ratio: 2:1

¾ pound ground beef (25% fat)

¾ cup grated Parmesan cheese

½ cup almond flour

1 large egg

¼ sweet onion, minced

1 teaspoon minced garlic

1 teaspoon dried basil

½ teaspoon dried oregano

Pinch ground allspice

2 tablespoons extra-virgin olive oil

IN MENU FOR WEEK:

3

Simple Reuben Casserole

SERVES 4 / PREP TIME: 25 MINUTES / COOK TIME: 20 MINUTES

Butter, for greasing

½ pound corned beef, diced

1 (32-ounce) jar sauerkraut, drained

1 cup shredded Swiss cheese, divided

8 ounces cream cheese, softened

½ teaspoon caraway seeds

One Pot • Make Ahead *The traditional Reuben sandwich consists of corned beef or pastrami, Swiss cheese, and sauerkraut. Sauerkraut is a tangy fermented cabbage that has gained a great deal of attention as an important addition to a diet requiring probiotic foods to improve digestion. It can also help reduce inflammation, boost the immune system, and support heart health.*

1. Preheat the oven to 350°F.

2. Lightly butter an 8-cup casserole dish, and set aside.

3. In a large bowl, stir together the corned beef, sauerkraut, and ½ cup of the Swiss cheese.

4. Stir in the cream cheese and caraway seeds.

5. Spoon the mixture into the baking dish, and sprinkle the reserved ½ cup of cheese evenly on top.

6. Bake until the mixture is bubbling and the cheese is melted, about 20 minutes.

7. Serve.

PER SERVING: CALORIES: 436 / FAT: 34G / TOTAL CARBS: 12G
FIBER: 7G / NET CARBS: 5G / SUGAR: 4G / PROTEIN: 21G

Fat 70% / Carbs 10% / Protein 20%   Ratio: 2:1

Beef Stroganoff

SERVES 4 / PREP TIME: 20 MINUTES / COOK TIME: 30 MINUTES

One Pot *When deciding which cut of beef to use in this recipe, consider grass-fed beef if it suits your budget because it is lower in cholesterol and higher in beta-carotene and lutein than commercially raised animals. The creamy stroganoff sauce is exceptionally thick and rich, which makes it perfect if you serve this dish over mashed cauliflower or zucchini noodles. If you are going to freeze this dish, omit the sour cream because it will make the sauce grainy when you thaw it out again.*

1. In a large skillet over medium-high heat, heat the olive oil.

2. Sauté the beef until lightly browned, about 2 minutes.

3. Using a slotted spoon, remove the beef from the skillet and set aside on a plate.

4. Add the onion and garlic to the skillet, and sauté until the vegetables are softened, about 3 minutes.

5. Stir in the mushrooms, and sauté until they are lightly browned, about 5 minutes.

6. Add the beef broth, cream, and the beef with any accumulated juices.

7. Bring the mixture to a boil, reduce the heat to low, and simmer until the beef is very tender, about 15 minutes.

8. Stir in the sour cream and parsley, season with salt and pepper, and serve.

PER SERVING: CALORIES: 410 / FAT: 31G / TOTAL CARBS: 6G
FIBER: 1G / NET CARBS: 5G / SUGAR: 2G / PROTEIN: 29G

Fat 69% / Carbs 3% / Protein 28%   Ratio: 1:1

2 tablespoons extra-virgin olive oil

¾ pound top sirloin steak, cut into thin strips

1 sweet onion, chopped

2 teaspoons minced garlic

1 cup sliced button mushrooms

1 cup beef broth

1 cup heavy (whipping) cream

½ cup sour cream

2 tablespoons chopped fresh parsley

Sea salt

Freshly ground black pepper

IN MENU FOR WEEK:

4

A CLOSER LOOK: *Mushrooms are not grown in manure and they are pasteurized so cleaning them is a simple process. The best method is to wipe traces of soil or moss off the caps with a soft cloth and trim any woody ends off. Do not ever soak fresh mushrooms because this will reduce their shelf life.*

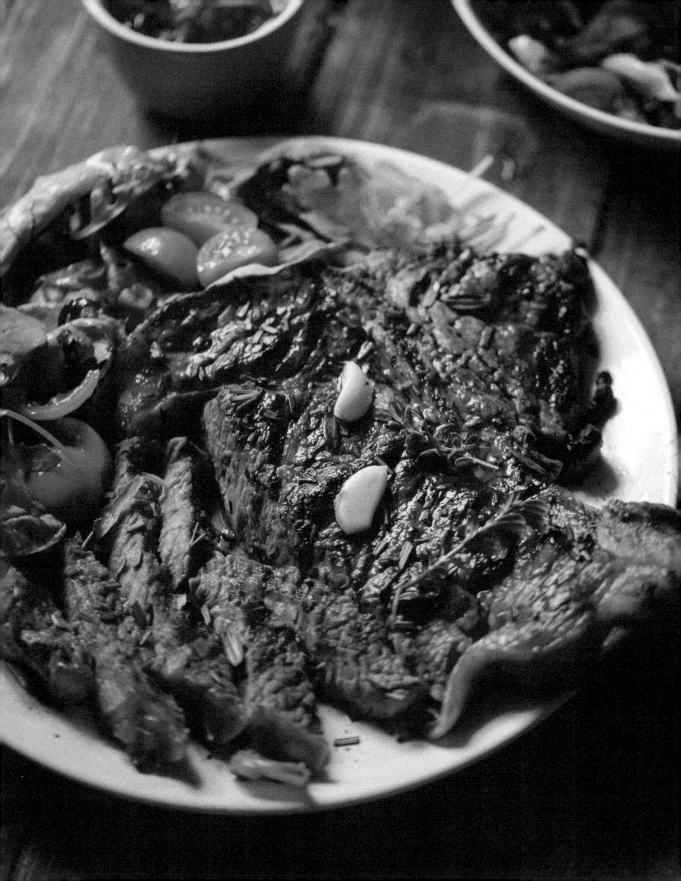

Rib Eye Steaks with Garlic-Thyme Butter

SERVES 4 / PREP TIME: 15 MINUTES, PLUS 30 MINUTES TO MARINATE / COOK TIME: 10 MINUTES

You can add other toppings to this simple steak depending on the occasion and your palate. Compound butters, creamy blue cheese sauce, or buttery sautéed mushrooms can create lovely variations.

1. Preheat the barbecue or grill pan to medium-high.

2. Rub the steaks all over with the olive oil, and season the meat on both sides with salt and pepper. Set aside for 30 minutes at room temperature.

3. Grill the steaks for 4 minutes per side for medium rare, or until desired doneness is reached.

4. Remove the steaks to a plate, and let them rest for 10 minutes.

5. While the steaks are resting, in a small skillet over medium-high heat, melt the butter.

6. Sauté the garlic and thyme for 2 minutes.

7. Top the steaks topped with the butter sauce and serve.

4 (6-ounce) rib eye steaks, about 1 inch thick

2 tablespoons extra-virgin olive oil

Sea salt

Freshly ground black pepper

2 tablespoons salted butter

2 teaspoons minced garlic

2 teaspoons chopped fresh thyme

IN MENU FOR WEEK:

2

PER SERVING: CALORIES: 581 / FAT: 45G / TOTAL CARBS: 2G
FIBER: 0G / NET CARBS: 2G / SUGAR: 0G / PROTEIN: 30G

Fat 76% / Carbs 1% / Protein 23%   Ratio: 2:1

Venison Pot Roast

SERVES 4 / PREP TIME: 15 MINUTES / COOK TIME: 2 HOURS 10 MINUTES

1 pound venison roast

Sea salt

**Freshly ground
black pepper**

¼ cup extra-virgin olive oil

1 celery stalk, chopped

**½ cup chopped
sweet onion**

1 teaspoon minced garlic

1 cup beef broth

2 bay leaves

1 teaspoon dried thyme

A CLOSER LOOK: *Celery
adds a slightly salty taste to
food, especially if you use
the greens. It is an excellent
source of vitamins A, B,
and C as well as potassium,
sodium, calcium, and iron.
Celery can protect against
neurological disease, cancer,
and cardiovascular disease.*

One Pot *Venison is no longer a meat that can only be enjoyed if
you hunt or know someone who does. Farmed venison is available in most grocery stores or butcher shops, and most of these
animals graze and are pasture raised. Venison is very high in protein but lean, so you will have to add fat to the dish to create moist
meat. Leftover roast can be wonderful in a soup or stew.*

1. Preheat the oven to 275°F.

2. Season the roast with salt and pepper.

3. In a large, ovenproof skillet over medium-high heat,
   heat the olive oil.

4. Sear the roast on all sides until lightly browned, about
   5 minutes total. Remove the roast to a plate.

5. Add the celery, onion, and garlic to the skillet, and sauté
   until softened, about 3 minutes.

6. Return the roast to the skillet with any accumulated
   juices on the plate, and stir in the beef broth, bay leaves,
   and thyme.

7. Cook the roast in the oven for 2 hours, turning
   it occasionally.

8. Remove the skillet from the oven, and take out the
   bay leaves.

9. Let the roast rest for 10 minutes before serving it with
   the pan drippings.

PER SERVING: CALORIES: 342 / FAT: 20G / TOTAL CARBS: 2G
FIBER: 0G / NET CARBS: 2G / SUGAR: 1G / PROTEIN: 40G

Fat 53% / Carbs 2% / Protein 45%   Ratio: 1:2

Grilled Venison Loin with Dijon Cream Sauce

SERVES 4 / PREP TIME: 10 MINUTES, PLUS 2 HOURS TO MARINATE / COOK TIME: 15 MINUTES

You might find yourself eating this incredible sauce right out of the pot with a spoon, so make a little extra. Reducing the cream and mustard intensifies the taste, so do not substitute Dijon mustard for the grainy one or the sauce will end up too salty. The venison loin should be medium if you use the timing in the recipe, so if you want the meat medium-rare, you should reduce the cooking time by about 1 minute per side.

1. Season the venison all over with the salt and pepper.

2. In a small bowl, stir together the olive oil, thyme, and rosemary, and rub the meat all over with the oil mixture.

3. Place the meat in a sealed freezer bag, and refrigerate for 2 hours.

4. Preheat the barbecue or grill pan to medium-high.

5. In a medium saucepan over medium heat, bring the cream to a simmer. Reduce the heat to low, and simmer until the cream is reduced by half into a thick, creamy sauce, about 5 minutes.

6. Remove the cream from the heat, and stir in the mustard, vinegar, and chives. Grill the venison, 4 to 5 minutes per side, turning to get all the surfaces browned.

7. Let the meat rest for 10 minutes, and serve with the sauce.

1 pound venison loin, trimmed of all silver skin

Sea salt

Freshly ground black pepper

2 tablespoons extra-virgin olive oil

1 teaspoon chopped fresh thyme

½ teaspoon chopped fresh rosemary

1½ cups heavy (whipping) cream

2 tablespoons grainy mustard

½ teaspoon apple cider vinegar

1 teaspoon chopped fresh chives

IN MENU FOR WEEKS:

PER SERVING: CALORIES: 394 / FAT: 28G / TOTAL CARBS: 2G
FIBER: 0G / NET CARBS: 2G / SUGAR: 0G / PROTEIN: 34G

Fat 64% / Carbs 2% / Protein 34%   Ratio: 1:2

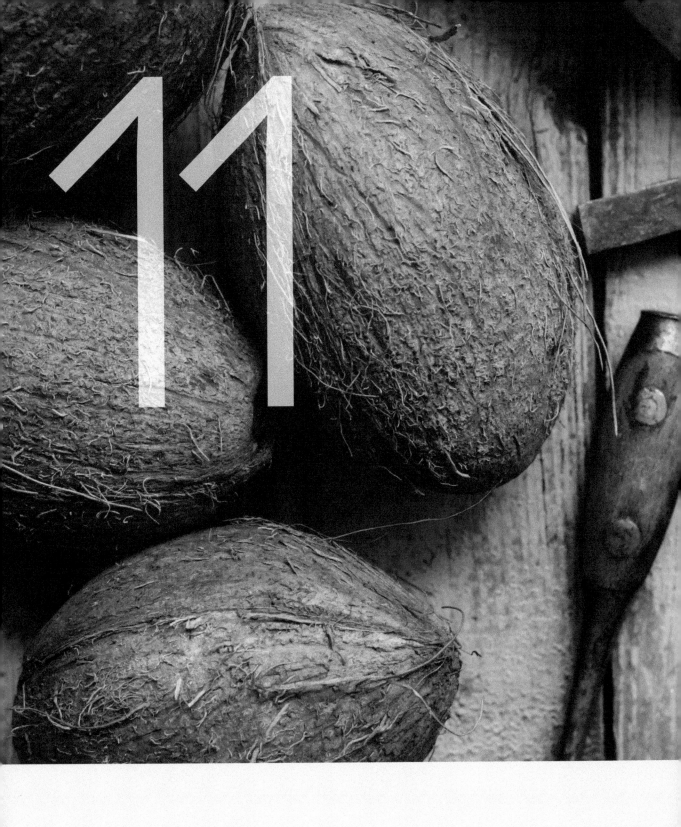

11

DESSERT

Chocolate-Chia Pudding

SERVES 4 / PREP TIME: 10 MINUTES, PLUS 6 HOURS TO SOAK

1 cup coconut milk

1 cup unsweetened almond milk

¼ cup chia seeds

¼ cup cocoa powder

2 tablespoons egg white protein powder

½ teaspoon stevia, or more

1 teaspoon pure vanilla extract

One Pot • Make Ahead *The texture of chia pudding is similar to tapioca; you can feel the tiny, liquid-plumped seeds on your tongue with every spoonful. If you are not a fan of the bumpy texture, you can create a pudding that is almost completely smooth with all the same health benefits. Just grind the chia seeds up to a powdery consistency in a blender, add the remaining ingredients, and pulse to combine. The pudding will be thick almost instantly, so you will not have to let it sit before eating.*

1. In a large bowl, stir together the coconut milk, almond milk, chia seeds, cocoa powder, egg white protein powder, stevia, and vanilla until well blended.

2. Refrigerate for at least 6 hours to soak.

3. Adjust the sweetness as desired, and serve.

PER SERVING: CALORIES: 226 / FAT: 18G / TOTAL CARBS: 10G
FIBER: 6G / NET CARBS: 4G / SUGAR: 2G / PROTEIN: 6G

Fat 71% / Carbs 18% / Protein 11%   Ratio: 3:1

Chocolate Parfaits

SERVES 4 / PREP TIME: 20 MINUTES

Under 30 Minutes • Make Ahead *Parfaits are happy; they look charming and whimsical, especially if you layer them perfectly in real parfait glasses. You can put as many layers as you like, as long as the chocolate and whipped cream do not mix and ruin the effect. If you crave a chocolate mousse presentation instead, fold the whipped cream into the chocolate mixture until it is completely incorporated.*

1. In a blender, blend the avocado, cocoa powder, egg white protein powder, water, ½ teaspoon of the stevia, cinnamon, and salt until the pudding is smooth and thick, adding more water as needed to adjust the texture. Set aside.

2. In a large bowl, whisk the heavy cream and the remaining ¼ teaspoon stevia until firm peaks form, about 5 minutes.

3. Set up 4 parfait or regular glasses.

4. Spoon 1 tablespoon of chocolate pudding into each of the glasses, and top each with 2 tablespoons of whipped cream. Repeat the layering until all the pudding is used up, and you end with whipped cream on the top.

5. Refrigerate the parfaits until you want to serve them.

1 avocado, peeled and pitted

¼ cup cocoa powder

¼ cup egg white protein powder

¼ cup water

¾ teaspoon stevia, divided

¼ teaspoon ground cinnamon

Pinch sea salt

1½ cups heavy (whipping) cream

PER SERVING: CALORIES: 280 / FAT: 24G / TOTAL CARBS: 9G
FIBER: 5G / NET CARBS: 4G / SUGAR: 1G / PROTEIN: 7G

Fat 75% / Carbs 13% / Protein 12%   Ratio: 3:1

Creamy Panna Cotta

SERVES 4 / PREP TIME: 20 MINUTES, PLUS 8 HOURS TO SET

1 tablespoon butter, softened, plus more for greasing

½ (7g) gelatin package

½ cup warm water

6 ounces cream cheese, softened

½ teaspoon pure vanilla extract

¼ teaspoon stevia

A CLOSER LOOK: *Gelatin not only provides the structure to create firm, velvety panna cotta, it also adds protein to this dessert. This handy ingredient is made from dried and powdered connective tissues, collagenous joints, and tendons of cows, pigs, and some fish. Including gelatin in your diet can improve your hair and skin as well as boost gut health.*

Make Ahead *Plain panna cotta has a light taste, so traditionally this dessert was served with thick sauces, fresh fruit, or chocolate to make something more complex. Panna cotta means "cooked cream," and since this recipe has no cream in it, it is actually not a true panna cotta. The texture is almost identical, and it has a lovely vanilla tanginess that can be enjoyed with a spoon and good company. Try layering in a spoon of puréed strawberries or topping this creamy treat with fresh blueberries for an elegant presentation.*

1. Lightly grease 4 muffin cups with butter, and set aside.

2. In a small bowl, sprinkle the gelatin over the water, and set aside.

3. In a medium bowl, beat together the cream cheese and butter until very smooth.

4. Beat in the gelatin mixture, vanilla, and stevia until smooth.

5. Spoon the panna cotta mixture into the muffin cups, and refrigerate for about 8 hours to set.

6. Run a knife around the edges of the cups, and flip the muffin tray over to remove the panna cottas.

7. Flip them over, and serve.

PER SERVING: CALORIES: 194 / FAT: 18G / TOTAL CARBS: 2G
FIBER: 0G / NET CARBS: 2G / SUGAR: 0G / PROTEIN: 6G

Fat 83% / Carbs 5% / Protein 12%   Ratio: 3:1

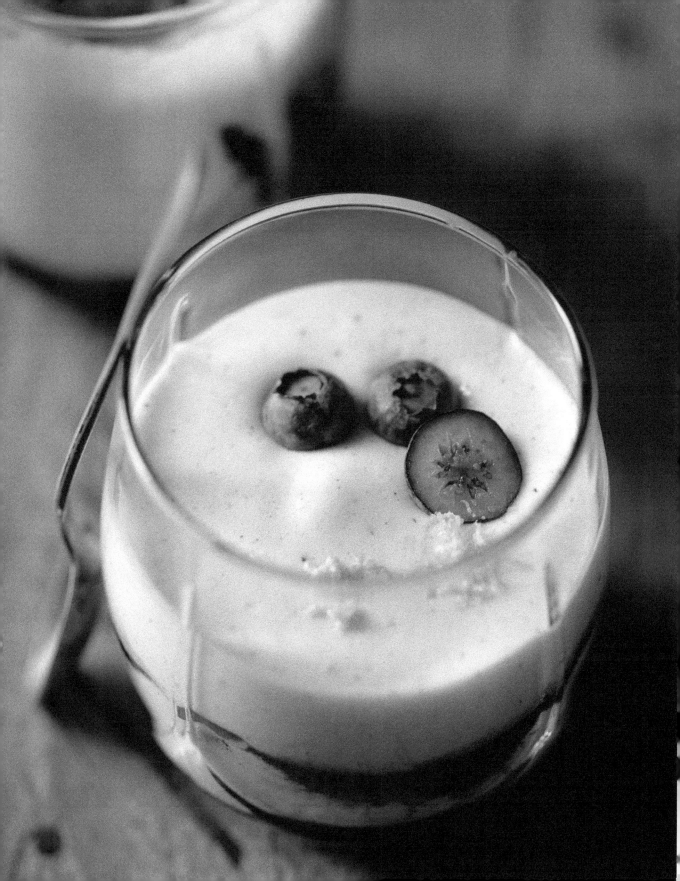

Sour Cream Ice Cream

SERVES 4 / PREP TIME: 10 MINUTES, PLUS FREEZING TIME

1 cup sour cream

1 cup unsweetened almond milk

3 tablespoons egg white protein powder

2 tablespoons freshly squeezed lemon juice

½ teaspoon stevia

½ teaspoon pure vanilla extract

TRY INSTEAD: *If you enjoy a good cheesecake, this ice cream might become your new favorite indulgence. Yogurt will work well in this recipe instead of sour cream, and a combination of 1 cup heavy cream and 1 teaspoon vinegar is also effective for a nice tangy flavor.*

Make Ahead *You do not need an ice cream maker to create ice cream, although the texture might not be as creamy as products created in an appliance. You can instead pour the ice cream mixture into a stainless steel baking dish, and place the dish in the freezer. Take the dish out every 30 minutes, and stir the mixture, scraping any frozen sections off the sides and bottom. Continue this process until the entire mixture is frozen, about 6 hours.*

1. In a blender, blend the sour cream, almond milk, egg white protein powder, lemon juice, stevia, and vanilla until smooth.

2. Transfer the mixture to an ice cream maker, and freeze according to the manufacturer's directions.

3. Serve.

PER SERVING: CALORIES: 149 / FAT: 13G / TOTAL CARBS: 3G
FIBER: 0G / NET CARBS: 3G / SUGAR: 0G / PROTEIN: 5G

Fat 77% / Carbs 9% / Protein 14%   Ratio: 3:1

Elegant Fudge Ice Pops

SERVES 4 / PREP TIME: 15 MINUTES, PLUS 3 HOURS TO FREEZE / COOK TIME: 1 MINUTE

Make Ahead *If there is such a thing as adult Popsicles, these fudgy beauties should meet the guidelines. The chocolate used is dark, so the flavor is not too sweet, and the color is deep brown. If you want a more kid-friendly version, use milk chocolate, white chocolate, or semi-sweet to create a less intense taste. Mini chocolate chips are also a good addition to the ice pops.*

1. In a small, microwave-safe bowl, microwave the chocolate and coconut oil on low power, watching carefully, until the chocolate is melted, about 1 minute.

2. Stir, and set aside.

3. In a blender, purée the avocado, almond milk, egg white protein powder, cocoa, stevia, and vanilla until the mixture is smooth.

4. Pour the coconut oil mixture into the blender, and blend until well incorporated.

5. Evenly divide the chocolate mixture among 4 ice pop molds.

6. Place the molds in the freezer and freeze, about 3 hours.

7. Serve.

1 ounce unsweetened chocolate

1 tablespoon coconut oil

½ avocado

½ cup unsweetened almond milk

2 tablespoons egg white protein powder

1 tablespoon cocoa powder

½ teaspoon stevia

½ teaspoon pure vanilla extract

PER SERVING: CALORIES: 144 / FAT: 12G / TOTAL CARBS: 5G
FIBER: 3G / NET CARBS: 2G / SUGAR: 0G / PROTEIN: 4G

Fat 75% / Carbs 14% / Protein 11%   Ratio: 3:1

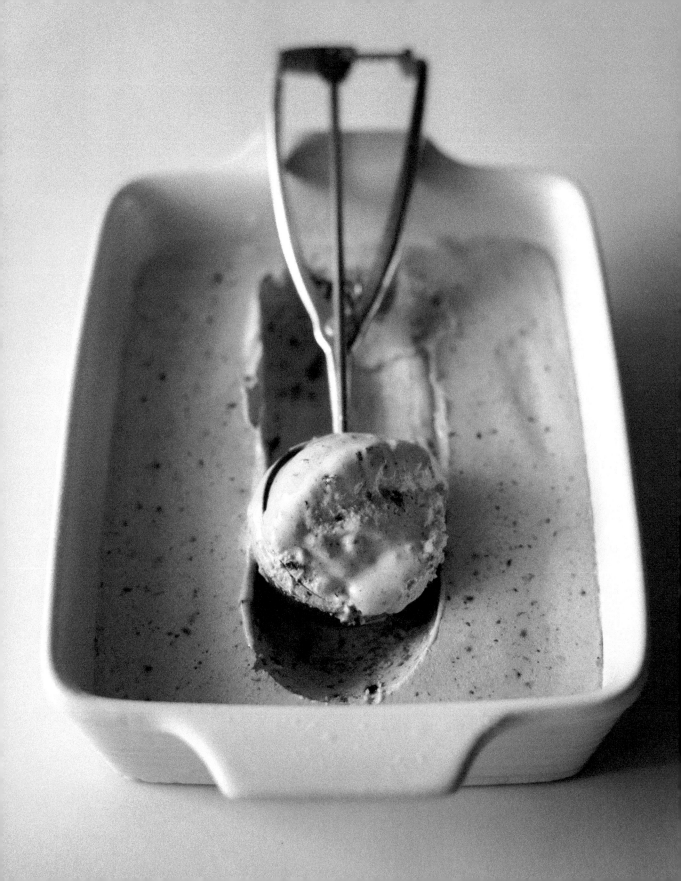

Strawberry Frozen Yogurt

MAKES 3 CUPS / PREP TIME: 10 MINUTES, PLUS FREEZING TIME

Make Ahead *Frozen yogurt is considered a healthier option for dessert than standard ice cream, especially if you make it from scratch. This recipe ends up pale pink with flecks of strawberry in the mix. If you like chunks of berry, only blend up half the berries, and then stir in the rest before freezing. The bar on the ice cream maker will break the berries up a bit more, but leave enough big pieces to be visible when you scoop up the dessert.*

1. In a blender, pulse the coconut milk, yogurt, strawberries, egg white protein powder, coconut oil, and stevia until the mixture is well blended and the strawberries are chopped.

2. Transfer the mixture to an ice cream maker, and freeze according to the manufacturer's directions.

3. Serve.

PER SERVING (¾ CUP): CALORIES: 140 / FAT: 12G / TOTAL CARBS: 4G
FIBER: 1G / NET CARBS: 3G / SUGAR: 3G / PROTEIN: 4G

Fat 76% / Carbs 12% / Protein 12%   Ratio: 3:1

1 cup coconut milk

1 cup plain Greek yogurt

½ cup sliced strawberries

3 tablespoons egg white protein powder

2 tablespoons coconut oil

½ teaspoon stevia

TRY INSTEAD: *Any type of berry or a combination of berries can be substituted for the strawberries in this ice cream. Raspberries and blackberries can be used in equal amounts to the strawberries, but the total carbohydrate amount will double per serving if you use blueberries.*

Fluffy Lime-Meringue Clouds

SERVES 4 / PREP TIME: 30 MINUTES / COOK TIME: 3 HOURS

FOR THE MERINGUES
4 large egg whites

½ teaspoon stevia

1 teaspoon pure vanilla extract

FOR THE LIME CURD
2 large eggs

2 teaspoons lime zest

¼ teaspoon stevia

¼ cup freshly squeezed lime juice

3 tablespoons coconut oil

FOR THE TOPPING
1 cup heavy (whipping) cream

KITCHEN HACK: *If you own a cake-decorating piping bag and star tip, you can pipe out truly lovely meringues instead of simple indented boats. Fill the piping bag with the meringue, and create disks in the correct size on your parchment paper; then pipe two layers around the sides to create a pretty ridged container.*

Meringues are an almost zero-calorie container for fillings and fruit that also have a reasonable amount of protein. The oven temperature is the key to meringues because you want to very slowly dry them out with absolutely no color change. This process takes time, and even a small heat increase can brown the egg white mixture, which is not the hallmark of this dessert. If you can spare your oven, turn it off after the meringues are done and leave the baking tray in the oven overnight to dry even more.

TO MAKE THE MERINGUES

1. Preheat the oven to 200°F.

2. Cover a baking sheet with parchment paper, and set aside.

3. In a large bowl, beat together the egg whites, stevia, and vanilla until the whites form stiff peaks, about 8 minutes.

4. Scoop the egg whites onto the baking sheet to form 4 mounds, and make a well in the center of each mound to create a bowl.

5. Bake the meringues in the oven until they are crisp and set, about 3 hours.

TO MAKE THE LIME CURD

1. While the meringues are baking, in a small saucepan over medium heat, whisk the eggs, lime zest, and stevia until the eggs are pale and slightly thickened, about 3 minutes.

2. Whisk in the lime juice and coconut oil until the mixture starts to bubble, about 5 minutes. Remove the saucepan from the heat.

3. Strain the curd through a fine mesh sieve into a small bowl.

4. Cover the top of the curd with plastic wrap, pressing the plastic right to the surface of the curd, and refrigerate until completely cooled.

TO MAKE THE TOPPING

1. In a medium bowl, beat the cream until it forms soft peaks.

2. Place 1 meringue on each plate, and evenly divide the lime curd among the meringues.

3. Top the dessert with the whipped cream, and serve.

PER SERVING: CALORIES: 260 / FAT: 24G / TOTAL CARBS: 3G
FIBER: 0G / NET CARBS: 3G / SUGAR: 1G / PROTEIN: 8G

Fat 82% / Carbs 5% / Protein 13%   Ratio: 3:1

Lemon Cheesecake

SERVES 4 / PREP TIME: 30 MINUTES, PLUS 1 HOUR TO SET

1 (7g) gelatin package

¼ cup heavy (whipping) cream

8 ounces cream cheese, softened

2 tablespoons freshly squeezed lemon juice

1 teaspoon stevia

1 teaspoon pure vanilla extract

One Pot • Make Ahead *Unbaked cheesecakes are often almost bouncy in their texture because they contain too much gelatin for the ingredient ratio. Cheesecake should just set up and still have a slightly grainy texture of the cream cheese, not seem like creamy Jell-O. You can use sheet gelatin instead of granules, but getting the substitution ratio correct is difficult; it's about 3 sheets per packet.*

1. In a small bowl, sprinkle the gelatin over the heavy cream. Set aside for 10 minutes.

2. In a large bowl, beat the cream cheese with a hand beater until it is smooth and fluffy, about 4 minutes.

3. Beat in the lemon juice, stevia, and vanilla, scraping down the sides of the bowl at least once.

4. Add the cream mixture to the large bowl, and beat to blend.

5. Spoon the lemon cheesecake mixture into 4 small serving dishes, and chill until they are set, about 1 hour.

6. Serve.

PER SERVING: CALORIES: 235 / FAT: 23G / TOTAL CARBS: 2G
FIBER: 0G / NET CARBS: 2G / SUGAR: 0G / PROTEIN: 7G

Fat 84% / Carbs 4% / Protein 12%　　Ratio: 3:1

Almond Cake

SERVES 12 / PREP TIME: 15 MINUTES / COOK TIME: 60 MINUTES

Make Ahead *This versatile batter can also be baked into muffins or cupcakes for a rich, golden treat. Simply reduce the cooking time to about 30 minutes for the smaller baked goods. The batter can also be studded with berries and chopped nuts and topped with a buttery icing if you want a more elegant presentation. A Swiss meringue buttercream recipe can be modified with a sweetener instead of granulated sugar.*

1. Preheat the oven to 300°F.

2. Lightly grease a 9-by-4-inch loaf pan with butter, and set aside.

3. In a large bowl, stir together the almond flour, egg white protein powder, baking powder, baking soda, stevia, and salt.

4. In a medium bowl, whisk together the eggs, almond milk, yogurt, vanilla, and almond extract.

5. Add the wet ingredients to the dry ingredients, and stir to blend well.

6. Spoon the batter into the loaf pan, and smooth the top with a spatula.

7. Bake until the loaf is golden and firm, about 60 minutes.

8. Cool the cake for 10 minutes in the pan, and then flip it out to cool completely on a wire rack.

9. Serve.

Butter, for greasing

2½ cups almond flour

½ cup egg white protein powder

2 teaspoons baking powder

1 teaspoon baking soda

1 teaspoon stevia

¼ teaspoon sea salt

3 large eggs

½ cup almond milk

½ cup plain Greek yogurt

1 teaspoon pure vanilla extract

1 teaspoon almond extract

PER SERVING (1 SLICE): CALORIES: 198 / FAT: 16G / TOTAL CARBS: 6G
FIBER: 3G / NET CARBS: 3G / SUGAR: 2G / PROTEIN: 5G

Fat 73% / Carbs 14% / Protein 13%   Ratio: 3:1

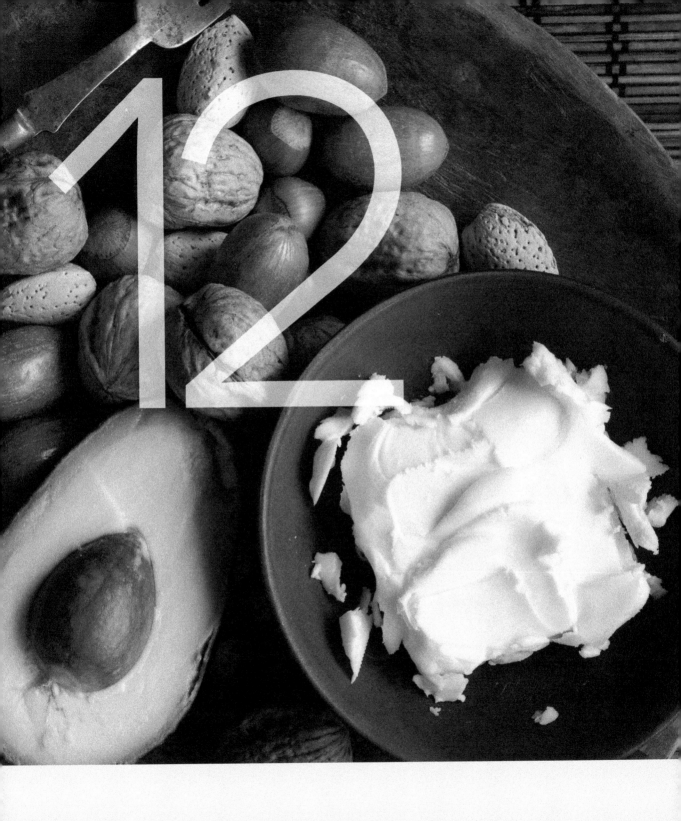

KITCHEN STAPLES

Buttermilk Ranch Dressing

MAKES 1½ CUPS / PREP TIME: 10 MINUTES

½ cup heavy (whipping) cream

1 teaspoon apple cider vinegar

½ cup Mayonnaise (page 213)

¼ cup sour cream

1 tablespoon freshly squeezed lemon juice

2 tablespoons chopped fresh parsley

2 tablespoons chopped fresh chives

½ teaspoon minced garlic

¼ teaspoon ground cayenne pepper

Sea salt

Freshly ground black pepper

Under 30 Minutes • Make Ahead *There is no buttermilk in this recipe, but the acidic cider vinegar added to the cream creates a very similar taste. Real buttermilk has 3 times the amount of carbs as heavy cream—about 2 grams to 6 grams in a ½-cup portion. Buttermilk is also lower in fat and protein than heavy cream and so is less appropriate for the keto lifestyle.*

1. In a small bowl, stir together the heavy cream and apple cider vinegar, and set aside for 10 minutes.

2. In a medium bowl, whisk together the Mayonnaise, sour cream, lemon juice, parsley, chives, garlic, cayenne pepper, and the reserved cream mixture until very well blended.

3. Season the dressing with salt and pepper.

4. Store the dressing in the refrigerator for up to 1 week.

PER SERVING (2 TABLESPOONS): CALORIES: 74 / FAT: 6G
TOTAL CARBS: 3G / FIBER: 0G / NET CARBS: 3G
SUGAR: 1G / PROTEIN: 2G

Fat 73% / Carbs 16% / Protein 11%   Ratio: 3:1

Traditional Caesar Dressing

MAKES 1 CUP / PREP TIME: 15 MINUTES

Under 30 Minutes • One Pot • Make Ahead *Raw eggs add to the rich emulsion of this classic dressing, but even pasteurized yolks should not be used if you are serving this to pregnant women, young children, or anyone whose health is compromised. Try using eggs from pasture-raised birds because there have never been any food poisoning incidents reported from those products. If you are still concerned, you can substitute 3 teaspoons of home-made Mayonnaise (page 213) for the yolks.*

1. In a blender, blend the anchovies, garlic, egg yolks, lemon juice, and Dijon mustard until the ingredients form a uniform paste.

2. Slowly drizzle the olive oil into the blender, while it is running, until the dressing is thick and emulsified and the oil is all gone.

3. Transfer the dressing to a container, and stir in the Parmesan cheese.

4. Season the dressing with salt and pepper.

5. Store the dressing in a sealed container in the fridge for up to 1 week.

PER SERVING (1 TABLESPOON): CALORIES: 80 / FAT: 8G
TOTAL CARBS: 0G / FIBER: 0G / NET CARBS: 0G
SUGAR: 0G / PROTEIN: 2G

Fat 90% / Carbs 0% / Protein 10%   Ratio: 4:1

5 anchovy fillets packed in oil, drained

2 garlic cloves

3 large pasteurized egg yolks

2 tablespoons freshly squeezed lemon juice

1 teaspoon Dijon mustard

½ cup extra-virgin olive oil

¼ cup grated Parmesan cheese

Sea salt

Freshly ground black pepper

A CLOSER LOOK: *Anchovies, not a commonly used fish in North America, are usually only seen in this dressing and on pizza. Anchovies are a small fish with tiny scales and edible, thin skin. The anchovies used in Caesar dressing are not fresh but jarred in oil or cured and tinned.*

Lemon-Garlic Dressing

MAKES 1 CUP / PREP TIME: 10 MINUTES

½ cup sour cream

¼ cup extra-virgin olive oil

1 tablespoon Dijon mustard

¼ cup freshly squeezed
lemon juice

2 teaspoons minced garlic

2 teaspoons chopped
fresh basil

2 teaspoons chopped
fresh parsley

2 teaspoons chopped
fresh thyme

Sea salt

Freshly ground
black pepper

Under 30 Minutes • One Pot • Make Ahead *Salads, steamed vegetables, baked fish, and crudités can all benefit from a little of this herb-infused, sour cream–based dressing. You might not realize that leaving heavy cream out at room temperature to ferment and thicken, creating sour cream, has been around for centuries. As the demand grew for this tangy dairy product, the production time was sped up with thickeners, such as gelatin, and added acids. Commercially produced sour cream is less healthy than natural products and contains less fat.*

1. In a medium bowl, whisk together the sour cream, olive oil, Dijon mustard, lemon juice, garlic, basil, parsley, and thyme until well blended.

2. Season the dressing with salt and pepper.

3. Transfer the dressing to a container and store, sealed, in the refrigerator for up to 1 week.

PER SERVING (2 TABLESPOONS): CALORIES: 98 / FAT: 10G
TOTAL CARBS: 1G / FIBER: 0G / NET CARBS: 1G
SUGAR: 0G / PROTEIN: 1G

Fat 92% / Carbs 4% / Protein 4%   Ratio: 10:1

Mayonnaise

MAKES 2 CUPS / PREP TIME: 5 MINUTES

Under 30 Minutes • One Pot • Make Ahead *If you use a lot of mayonnaise, you might want to double the recipe. An immersion (handheld) blender can be used to create mayonnaise in less than a minute. Put the egg, mustard, and lemon juice in a large glass or jar, and purée for about 15 seconds to blend. Add the olive oil, and blend until the mayonnaise is thick and creamy, about 30 seconds. Season with salt and pepper, and store the mayo in the refrigerator.*

1. In a medium bowl, whisk together the egg and Dijon mustard until very well blended, about 2 minutes.

2. Add the olive oil in a continuous thin stream, whisking constantly, until the mayonnaise is thick and completely emulsified.

3. Whisk in the lemon juice.

4. Season with salt and pepper.

5. Store the mayonnaise in the fridge in an airtight container for up to 4 days.

1 large egg

1 tablespoon Dijon mustard

¾ cup extra-virgin olive oil

2 tablespoons freshly squeezed lemon juice

Sea salt

Freshly ground black pepper

KITCHEN HACK: *The lemon juice in this recipe adds a perfect sour finish and whitens the mayonnaise. If you want to save time, use bottled lemon juice instead of squeezing your own.*

PER SERVING (2 TABLESPOONS): CALORIES: 94 / FAT: 10G
TOTAL CARBS: 0G / FIBER: 0G / NET CARBS: 0G
SUGAR: 0G / PROTEIN: 1G

Fat 96% / Carbs 0% / Protein 4%   Ratio: 10:1

Herbed Marinara Sauce

SERVES 4 / PREP TIME: 10 MINUTES

1 (14-ounce) can
unsweetened
whole tomatoes

2 tablespoons extra-virgin
olive oil

2 tablespoons grated
Parmesan cheese

1 tablespoon balsamic
vinegar

1 teaspoon chopped
fresh basil

1 teaspoon chopped
fresh oregano

1 teaspoon chopped
fresh parsley

Pinch red pepper flakes

Pinch sea salt

Pinch freshly ground
black pepper

Under 30 Minutes • One Pot • Make Ahead *You might have
thought rich tomato sauces were off your menu when starting
the keto lifestyle, so this recipe might be a nice surprise. There
are still tomatoes as the base of the sauce, and the carbs are
slightly higher than you might want; however, when combined
with other foods such as breaded chicken and mozzarella cheese
(Chicken Parmigiana), the percentages of fat, protein, and carbs
are perfect.*

1. In a food processor, pulse the tomatoes, olive oil,
   Parmesan cheese, vinegar, basil, oregano, parsley,
   red pepper flakes, sea salt, and pepper until the sauce
   is smooth.

2. Store the sauce in a sealed container in the fridge
   until you want to use it, and then heat the sauce in a
   saucepan over low heat.

PER SERVING (½ CUP): CALORIES: 96 / FAT: 8G / TOTAL CARBS: 4G
FIBER: 2G / NET CARBS: 2G / SUGAR: 2G / PROTEIN: 2G

Fat 75% / Carbs 17% / Protein 8%   Ratio: 4:1

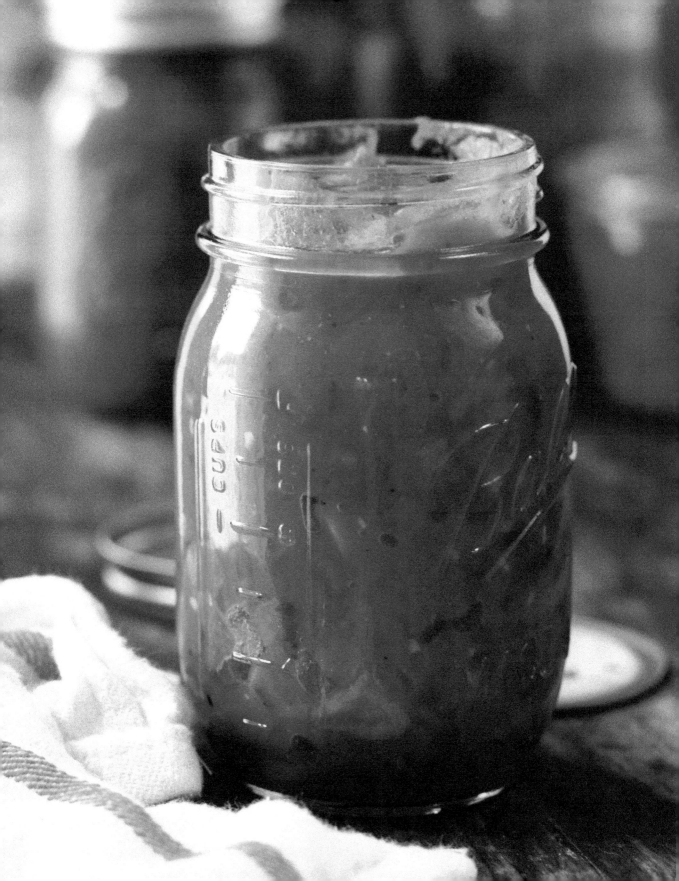

Indonesian Peanut Sauce

MAKES 2 CUPS / PREP TIME: 5 MINUTES

1 cup natural peanut butter

¼ cup toasted sesame oil

¼ cup freshly squeezed lemon juice

2 tablespoons tahini

1 tablespoon soy sauce

½ teaspoon red pepper flakes

¼ teaspoon stevia

Water, for thinning

TRY INSTEAD: *Any type of nut butter such as almond butter, cashew butter, or hazelnut butter can replace the peanut butter in this fiery sauce. The taste will change slightly, but it will still be delicious and combine well with the other ingredients.*

Under 30 Minutes • One Pot • Make Ahead *Peanuts are not actually nuts; they are a nutrient-packed legume that are roasted and ground up for nut butter. Peanuts are extremely rich in heart-friendly monounsaturated fats, vitamin E, protein, and manganese. Peanuts also have one of the highest antioxidant profiles of any food, which means they protect against cancer and Alzheimer's disease, and can lower the risk of obesity.*

1. In a blender, blend the peanut butter, sesame oil, lemon juice, tahini, soy sauce, red pepper flakes, and stevia until very smooth.

2. Thin the sauce with water if you want a thinner consistency.

3. Store the sauce in a sealed container in the refrigerator for up to 1 week.

PER SERVING (2 TABLESPOONS): CALORIES: 147 / FAT: 13G
TOTAL CARBS: 4G / FIBER: 1G / NET CARBS: 3G
SUGAR: 1G / PROTEIN: 6G

Fat 77% / Carbs 8% / Protein 15%   Ratio: 2:1

Garlicky Alfredo Sauce

SERVES 8 / PREP TIME: 15 MINUTES / COOK TIME: 12 MINUTES

Under 30 Minutes • One Pot *You will not need very much of this sauce for each portion, about ½ cup, because it is so rich and creamy. Toss the Alfredo sauce with zucchini noodles, spoon the sauce over chicken or pork, or drizzle a little over steamed cauliflower or broccoli for a quick side dish. You can use Parmesan cheese instead of Asiago if you prefer the taste or do not use Asiago regularly in your recipes.*

¼ cup butter

2 tablespoons minced sweet onion

2 teaspoons minced garlic

2 large egg yolks

1 cup heavy (whipping) cream

1½ cups freshly grated Asiago cheese

1 teaspoon chopped fresh basil

Sea salt

Freshly ground black pepper

1. In a large saucepan over medium heat, melt the butter.

2. Sauté the onion and garlic until softened, about 3 minutes.

3. Whisk in the egg yolks and cream.

4. Bring the sauce to a boil, and reduce the heat to low so that it simmers and thickens, about 5 minutes.

5. Whisk in the cheese and basil, and simmer for 2 minutes.

6. Season the sauce with salt and pepper, and serve over chicken or vegetables.

PER SERVING (½ CUP): CALORIES: 186 / FAT: 18G / TOTAL CARBS: 1G
FIBER: 0G / NET CARBS: 0G / SUGAR: 0G / PROTEIN: 6G

Fat 87% / Carbs 0% / Protein 13%   Ratio: 3:1

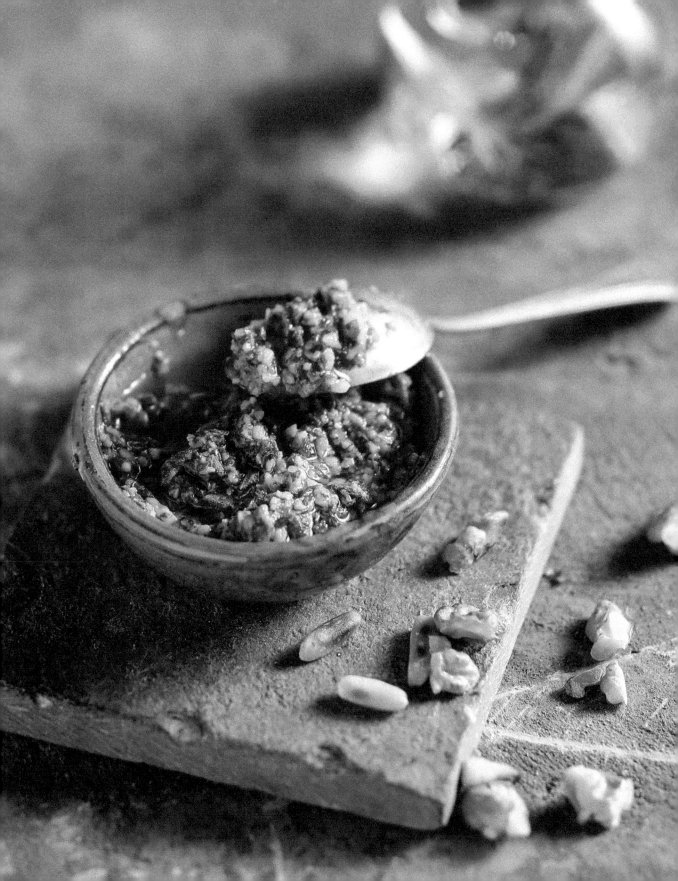

Herb Pesto

MAKES 2 CUPS / PREP TIME: 15 MINUTES

Under 30 Minutes • One Pot • Make Ahead *You might have fresh herbs left over after making pesto because the bunches are quite large and the amount needed is not substantial. Freezing extra herbs is a fabulous method to preserve them for another recipe. Some of the best herbs that benefit from freezing include the ones in this recipe and others such as parsley, dill, fennel greens, tarragon, chives, chervil, and lemon balm. Spread whole or chopped herbs in a single layer on trays, and place trays in the freezer for about 10 minutes, then remove trays from the freezer and transfer frozen herbs to labeled, sealable freezer bags or plastic containers.*

1 cup fresh basil

½ cup fresh oregano

½ cup fresh mint

¼ cup freshly squeezed lemon juice

½ cup walnuts

1 clove garlic

1 cup extra-virgin olive oil

1. In a blender, pulse the basil, oregano, mint, lemon juice, walnuts, and garlic clove until the mixture is very finely chopped.
2. Drizzle in the olive oil in a thin stream while the blender is running until all the oil is used up.
3. Scrape down the sides of the blender, and pulse until the pesto is uniform.
4. Store the pesto in a sealed container in the refrigerator up to 2 weeks.

TRY INSTEAD: *Basil pesto is the standard product that lines grocery shelves, but any herb or dark leafy green can be used in this recipe with fabulous results. Kale, spinach, thyme, cilantro, and summer savory all create fragrant, vibrantly green pesto, which can be used for many different recipes.*

PER SERVING (1 TABLESPOON): CALORIES: 72 / FAT: 8G
TOTAL CARBS: 1G / FIBER: 1G / NET CARBS: 0G
SUGAR: 0G / PROTEIN: 1G

Fat 88% / Carbs 6% / Protein 6%   Ratio: 8:1

Hollandaise

MAKES 1 CUP / PREP TIME: 20 MINUTES / COOK TIME: 20 MINUTES

¾ cup unsalted butter

2 large egg yolks

1 teaspoon cold water

Juice of ½ lemon, about
2 teaspoons

Pinch sea salt

Hollandaise is the buttery, decadent sauce that is poured over eggs Benedict in fancy restaurants, all the more opulent because this sauce will not hold much longer than a couple of hours. Sometimes, despite your best efforts, the hollandaise sauce you worked so hard on might break or separate. If this happens, whisk in about 1 to 2 teaspoons of boiling water a few drops at a time. When all else fails, whisk in another yolk until the sauce stays together again.

1. In a medium saucepan over low heat, melt the butter.

2. Remove the saucepan from the heat, and let the melted butter stand for 10 minutes.

3. Skim the foam from the top of the melted butter, and pour the clear yellow clarified part of the butter into a container; discard the milk solids.

4. Fill a medium saucepan over medium heat with about 3 inches of water.

5. When the water simmers gently, add the egg yolks and water to a large, stainless steel bowl, and whisk until they are foamy and light, about 3 minutes.

6. Add ½ teaspoon of lemon juice to the yolks, and whisk for about 1 minute.

7. Place the bowl onto the mouth of the saucepan, making sure the bottom of the bowl does not touch the simmering water.

8. Whisk the yolks until they thicken, about 2 minutes, and remove the bowl from the simmering water.

9. Pour the clarified butter in a very thin stream into the yolk mixture, whisking continuously, until you have used up all the butter and the sauce is thick and smooth.

10. Whisk in the remaining 1½ teaspoons of lemon juice, and season the sauce with salt.

11. Use the sauce immediately.

PER SERVING (2 TABLESPOONS): CALORIES: 166 / FAT: 18G / TOTAL CARBS: 0G
FIBER: 0G / NET CARBS: 0G / SUGAR: 0G / PROTEIN: 1G

Fat 96% / Carbs 0% / Protein 4%   Ratio: 18:1

Horseradish Compound Butter

MAKES 24 (½-INCH) DISKS / PREP TIME: 7 MINUTES

1 cup butter, softened

½ cup coconut oil

1 teaspoon prepared horseradish

1 garlic clove

1 tablespoon fresh chopped basil

1 tablespoon fresh chopped oregano

½ teaspoon freshly ground black pepper

¼ teaspoon sea salt

KITCHEN HACK: *You can find fresh horseradish in the produce section of the grocery store, usually among the potatoes or garlic. Simply peel and grate your own horseradish for this easy butter, but reduce the amount to ½ teaspoon because fresh horseradish is very potent.*

Under 30 Minutes • One Pot • Make Ahead *Compound butters are one of the easiest methods to enhance meats, chicken, fish, and vegetables. What could be simpler than to slice off a piece of butter and place it on your steak or chicken breast so that the flavors slowly melt? The combination of ingredients mixed into the butter is not set in stone. You can add other herbs, roasted garlic, sun-dried tomatoes, spices, and hot peppers to the mix or create several compound butters to keep in your freezer.*

1. In a blender, pulse the butter, coconut oil, horseradish, garlic, basil, oregano, pepper, and salt until the ingredients are well blended.

2. Lay a double layer of plastic wrap, about 1 foot long, on a counter, and scoop the butter mixture onto the plastic lengthwise.

3. Fold the plastic wrap over the butter mixture, creating a long tube. Hold one end of the wrap firmly, and slowly twist the other end, creating a tight cylinder of butter about 1 inch in diameter. Twist the other end, and tuck both ends under.

4. Refrigerate or freeze the butter cylinder until it is very firm. Cut off a slice of butter whenever you want to top vegetables, fish, or a nice steak.

5. Store the butter in the freezer for up to 1 month.

PER SERVING (½-INCH DISK): CALORIES: 108 / FAT: 12G
TOTAL CARBS: 0G / FIBER: 0G / NET CARBS: 0G
SUGAR: 0G / PROTEIN: 0G

Fat 100% / Carbs 0% / Protein 0%   Ratio: 2:1

Cinnamon-Caramel Sauce

MAKES 1 CUP / PREP TIME: 2 MINUTES / COOK TIME: 10 MINUTES

Under 30 Minutes • One Pot • Make Ahead *Caramel is usually made from very few ingredients such as sugar, cream, and butter. Since plain granulated sugar has a great many carbs in it, this recipe uses brown butter to create the nutty taste and golden color. You can easily double this recipe and use the sauce over desserts, in smoothies to add flavor, and for extra fat if you need to tweak your daily percentages.*

1. In a large saucepan over low heat, cook the butter until it becomes light brown and nutty smelling, about 4 minutes.

2. Whisk in the cream, stevia, and cinnamon.

3. Bring the mixture to a simmer, stirring constantly.

4. Continue simmering until the sauce is thickened, about 2 minutes.

5. Remove the saucepan from the heat, and continue to stir for at least 5 minutes, so that the sauce does not separate.

6. Store the sauce in a sealed container in the fridge for up to 4 days.

PER SERVING (2 TABLESPOONS): CALORIES: 130 / FAT: 14G
TOTAL CARBS: 0G / FIBER: 0G / NET CARBS: 0G
SUGAR: 0G / PROTEIN: 1G

Fat 97% / Carbs 0% / Protein 3%   Ratio: 14:1

½ cup butter

½ cup heavy (whipping) cream

1 teaspoon stevia

¼ teaspoon ground cinnamon

IN MENU FOR WEEKS:

Pastry Cream

SERVES 6 / PREP TIME: 10 MINUTES, PLUS 2 HOURS TO CHILL / COOK TIME: 20 MINUTES

6 large egg yolks

3 cups unsweetened almond milk

½ teaspoon stevia

1 tablespoon arrowroot powder

1 teaspoon pure vanilla extract

1 tablespoon butter

IN MENU FOR WEEK:

3

TRY INSTEAD: *Arrowroot is a thickening agent that does not add any carbohydrates to this rich, creamy sauce. You can also use all-purpose flour or cornstarch, but they will add 1 gram of total carbs per serving to the sauce.*

Make Ahead *There is something luxurious about pastry cream; it is thick, creamy, and utterly luscious. You can use a couple spoonfuls for a filling in pies, spoon it over a plain cake, and drizzle a little over fruit. Pastry cream is even eaten as break-fast in some countries, such as the Netherlands, and since the calories are not too high, make a double portion, and enjoy it on a special morning.*

1. In a medium bowl, beat the egg yolks and almond milk until well blended.

2. Whisk the stevia and arrowroot together in a large saucepan, and gradually whisk in the milk mixture.

3. Over medium-low heat, cook, stirring constantly, until the mixture comes to a boil and thickens, about 20 minutes.

4. Remove the saucepan from the heat, and stir in the vanilla and butter.

5. Transfer the pastry cream to a medium bowl, and press a piece of plastic wrap on the surface of the pastry cream to prevent a skin from forming.

6. Place the pastry cream in the fridge until completely chilled, at least 2 hours.

PER SERVING (¾ CUP): CALORIES: 89 / FAT: 8G / TOTAL CARBS: 1G
FIBER: 1G / NET CARBS: 0G / SUGAR: 0G / PROTEIN: 4G

Fat 78% / Carbs 5% / Protein 17%   Ratio: 2:1

Coconut Pie Crust

MAKES 1 PIE CRUST / PREP TIME: 10 MINUTES / COOK TIME: 10 MINUTES

Under 30 Minutes • One Pot • Make Ahead *Making a good pie crust is the culinary quest of both professional and home cooks because it can be used for many recipes. This crust is not as flaky as a standard lard-and-flour creation, but the buttery crispness will satisfy even the most critical guest. You can omit the stevia if you are making this crust for quiche or a meat pie.*

½ cup butter, melted, plus more for greasing

3 large eggs

1 cup coconut flour

¼ teaspoon stevia

¼ teaspoon sea salt

1. Preheat the oven to 400°F.

2. Lightly grease a 10-inch pie pan with butter.

3. In a medium bowl, beat together the butter and eggs until blended.

4. Stir in the coconut flour, stevia, and salt with a fork so that the dough holds together.

5. Gather the dough into a ball, and press it into the pie plate.

6. Prick the entire surface with a fork.

7. Bake the crust until light brown, about 10 minutes.

8. Cool and fill.

PER SERVING (⅛ OF THE CRUST): CALORIES: 204 / FAT: 16G
TOTAL CARBS: 9G / FIBER: 6G / NET CARBS: 3G
SUGAR: 1G / PROTEIN: 6G

Fat 71% / Carbs 18% / Protein 11%   Ratio: 3:1

Bacon Chutney

MAKES 1½ CUPS / PREP TIME: 10 MINUTES / COOK TIME: 27 MINUTES

1 tablespoon coconut oil

½ pound bacon, chopped

1 sweet onion, diced

1 (14-ounce) can diced unsweetened tomatoes

½ teaspoon stevia

2 tablespoons apple cider vinegar

A CLOSER LOOK: *Apple cider vinegar is a health sensation linked to weight loss, lower blood sugar levels, and improved cardiovascular health. You can increase the amount in the recipe to create slightly tart chutney with no increase in carbs, fat, or protein.*

One Pot • Make Ahead *Chutneys are like hot salsa or relish with a little more sweetness and acid. Chutneys usually contain fruit, which is the role tomatoes play in this savory concoction. This condiment originated in India and was brought to England by returning expatriates in the seventeenth century. Chutney is wonderful on fish, meats, and chicken or as a tasty snack.*

1. In a large saucepan over medium heat, heat the coconut oil.

2. Cook the bacon until it is cooked through and crispy, about 4 minutes.

3. Using a slotted spoon, remove the bacon to a bowl, and set aside.

4. Sauté the onion until softened, about 3 minutes.

5. Add the tomatoes, reserved bacon, stevia, and vinegar to the saucepan.

6. Bring the mixture to a boil, reduce the heat to low, and simmer until the chutney is thick, about 20 minutes.

7. Spoon the chutney into a container, and let it cool before storing it, covered, in the refrigerator for up to 1 week.

PER SERVING (1 TABLESPOON): CALORIES: 62 / FAT: 5G
TOTAL CARBS: 1G / FIBER: 0G / NET CARBS: 0G
SUGAR: 1G / PROTEIN: 4G

Fat 75% / Carbs 5% / Protein 20%   Ratio: 1:1

Simple Egg Salad

MAKES 2 CUPS / PREP TIME: 15 MINUTES / COOK TIME: 8 MINUTES

Under 30 Minutes • Make Ahead *Eggs are a staple food in many homes because they can be used in any type of recipe, from breakfast to entrées and desserts. The way the chicken is raised and treated is important because it can affect the taste and quality of the eggs. Some of the best-tasting eggs are pasture raised from a reputable farmer, but try different eggs to find out which ones you like the best, taking into consideration cost, flavor, freshness, and how the birds are treated.*

8 large eggs

¼ cup Mayonnaise (page 213)

2 tablespoons coconut oil

½ teaspoon Dijon mustard

1 scallion, chopped

½ teaspoon freshly ground black pepper

¼ teaspoon sea salt

1. Place the eggs in the bottom of a large saucepan, in one layer, and cover the eggs with cold water by about 3 inches.

2. Place the saucepan over high heat, and bring to a boil.

3. Reduce the heat to medium, and boil the eggs for 8 minutes.

4. Remove the saucepan from the heat, and pour out the water. Run cold water over the eggs until they are cool to the touch.

5. Remove the eggs from the water, and peel them.

6. Grate the eggs into a medium bowl, and stir in the Mayonnaise, coconut oil, Dijon mustard, scallion, pepper, and salt.

7. Refrigerate until you are ready to eat.

PER SERVING (¼ CUP): CALORIES: 131 / FAT: 11G / TOTAL CARBS: 2G
FIBER: 0G / NET CARBS: 2G / SUGAR: 1G / PROTEIN: 6G

Fat 75% / Carbs 7% / Protein 18%   Ratio: 2:1

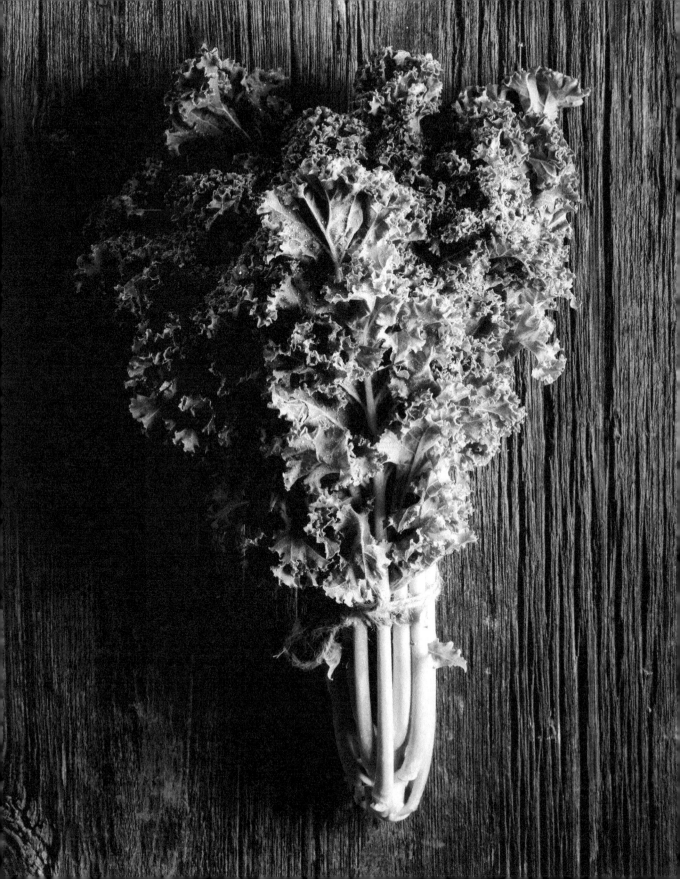

APPENDIX I: Conversion Tables

Volume Equivalents (Liquid)

US STANDARD	US STANDARD (OUNCES)	METRIC (APPROXIMATE)
2 tablespoons	1 fl. oz.	30 mL
¼ cup	2 fl. oz.	60 mL
½ cup	4 fl. oz.	120 mL
1 cup	8 fl. oz.	240 mL
1½ cups	12 fl. oz.	355 mL
2 cups or 1 pint	16 fl. oz.	475 mL
4 cups or 1 quart	32 fl. oz.	1 L
1 gallon	128 fl. oz.	4 L

Oven Temperatures

FAHRENHEIT (F)	CELSIUS (C) (APPROXIMATE)
250	120
300	150
325	165
350	180
375	190
400	200
425	220
450	230

Volume Equivalents (Dry)

US STANDARD	METRIC (APPROXIMATE)
⅛ teaspoon	0.5 mL
¼ teaspoon	1 mL
½ teaspoon	2 mL
¾ teaspoon	4 mL
1 teaspoon	5 mL
1 tablespoon	15 mL
¼ cup	59 mL
⅓ cup	79 mL
½ cup	118 mL
⅔ cup	156 mL
¾ cup	177 mL
1 cup	235 mL
2 cups or 1 pint	475 mL
3 cups	700 mL
4 cups or 1 quart	1 L
½ gallon	2 L
1 gallon	4 L

Weight Equivalents

US STANDARD	METRIC (APPROXIMATE)
½ ounce	15 g
1 ounce	30 g
2 ounces	60 g
4 ounces	115 g
8 ounces	225 g
12 ounces	340 g
16 ounces or 1 pound	455 g

Resources & Further Reading

Richoux, Celby. *Bacon & Butter*. Rockridge Press, Berkeley, CA. 2014.

Harvard Health Publications. "What You Eat Can Fuel or Cool Inflammation." September 1, 2005. www.health.harvard .edu/fhg/updates/What-you-eat-can -fuel-or-cool-inflammation-a-key-driver -of-heart-disease-diabetes-and-other -chronic-conditions.shtml.

Mancinelli, Kristen. *The Ketogenic Diet*. Ulysses Press, Berkeley, CA. 2015.

McKinley Health Center. "Breaking Down Your Metabolism." Accessed August 25, 2015. www.mckinley .illinois.edu/handouts/metabolism.htm.

Moore, Jimmy. *Keto Clarity*. Victory Belt Publishing, Riverside, NJ. 2014.

Slajerova, Martina. *The Keto Diet Blog*. Accessed August 25, 2015. ketodietapp.com/Blog.

Sondike SB, *et al.* "Effects of a low-carbohydrate diet on weight loss and cardiovascular risk factor in overweight adolescents." *The Journal of Pediatrics*, 2003.

Recipe Index

Index

CPSIA information can be obtained
at www.ICGtesting.com
Printed in the USA
LVHW01s2206270818
586068LV00001BA/1/P